THE
HEADACHE
GODFATHER

THE
HEADACHE
GODFATHER

*The Story of Dr. Seymour Diamond and How
He Revolutionized the Treatment of Headaches*

SEYMOUR DIAMOND, M.D.
CHARLIE MOREY

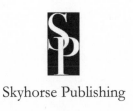

Skyhorse Publishing

Skyhorse Publishing books may be purchased in bulk at special discounts for sales promotion, corporate gifts, fund-raising, or educational purposes. Special editions can also be created to specifications. For details, contact the Special Sales Department, Skyhorse Publishing, 307 West 36th Street, 11th Floor, New York, NY 10018 or info@skyhorsepublishing.com.

Skyhorse® and Skyhorse Publishing® are registered trademarks of Skyhorse Publishing, Inc.®, a Delaware corporation.

Visit our website at www.skyhorsepublishing.com.

10 9 8 7 6 5 4 3 2 1

Library of Congress Cataloging-in-Publication Data is available on file.

Cover design by Qualcom Designs
Cover photo credit Linda Schwartz Photography

Print ISBN: 978-1-62914-538-9
Ebook ISBN: 978-1-62914-980-6

Printed in the United States of America

Dedications

To my grandchildren—Brian Diamond-Falk, Emily Diamond-Falk, Max Barack, Michael Diamond Barack, Jacob Barack, and Katelynn Barack—and to my great-grandchildren—Zevon and Oliver Diamond-Falk.

—Seymour Diamond

To my wife, Amy Diamond, who volunteered me for this project when she told her parents, "Charlie can write Dad's book!" and who's had confidence in me for everything I've ever attempted. And to headache sufferers around the world who have benefited from Seymour's efforts to ease their pain. As they'll learn from reading this book, it didn't come easily.

—Charlie Morey

Table of Contents

Foreword

> May there never develop in me the notion that my education is complete, but give me the strength and leisure and zeal, continually to enlarge my knowledge.
>
> —*Maimonides*

The life of Seymour Diamond, M.D., and his myriad accomplishments parallels the development of headache as a specialty and scientific pursuit. He arrived on the scene at the right time and with the right skills, and propelled the field of headache into the modern scientific era. His abilities are and were multidimensional: he revolutionized the care of the headache patient; he enlarged the armamentarium used in treating the headache patient; he created the settings in which care could be maximized; he revolutionized the approach to educating community physicians, specialists, and allied health personnel; he was a pioneer in patient and family education; and he energized the field of clinical research in headache. Dr. Diamond recognized the social, medical, financial, and emotional burden of headache long before his peers. In addition to all of the above skills, he brought his passion, his enormous energy, and his single-minded focus to the field of headache. These attributes allowed him to improve the lives of patients suffering with headache and decrease their disability—locally, nationally, and internationally.

To help the patient with disabling headache was his major focus. His innovations in this area are numerous. He was among the first to develop an outpatient clinic utilizing a multidisciplinary approach to treatment. Dr. Diamond recognized that some patients needed a more intensive treatment regimen, and he developed the premier hospital-based inpatient program recognizing that the most severely affected patients needed to be removed from their home setting and approached with a combination of emotional understanding, medications, treating withdrawal symptoms from narcotics, counseling, recreational therapy, physical therapy, and patient/family education. Indeed, this innovative approach to acute headache treatment brought relief to thousands. In order to accomplish this mission, he waged a constant battle with the "managed health care" companies. He proved that his innovative program was effective and cost-effective. His model is now recognized around the world as a necessary component in providing total care to the most resistant headache patients.

Dr. Diamond entered the area of pharmaceutical research with gusto. He saw this as a way to improve patient care. He partnered with companies to bring newer medications in a timely fashion to his patients. The earliest papers utilizing indomethacin, propranolol, and the tricyclic antidepressants to treat headache were authored by Dr. Diamond. His scientific investigations, his intellectual curiosity into the pathophysiology of headache, and his exploration of its clinical variation were pioneering. In addition, the clinical descriptions of unusual headache types were brought to the attention of fellow physicians by Dr. Diamond. Review of his curriculum vitae demonstrates hundreds of contributions to the literature advancing knowledge in the areas of patient care and pharmacology.

Dr. Diamond has always felt that his expertise needed wider dissemination in order to help a wider population of headache sufferers. His semiannual review courses for practicing physicians have impacted thousands of clinicians who brought newer medical advances home to their patients. His generosity with his time and experience is widely known. He helped found the National Headache Foundation, which enhances the dissemination of headache information to thousands of patients. He continues to work on behalf of the public, patients, and physicians to improve outcomes.

He was among the first of the adult headache specialists to recognize that "children were not little adults" and that their headaches were a specialized field of medicine. Dr. Diamond always included separate pediatric topics in his postgraduate courses. On a personal note, he inspired and encouraged me and my pediatric colleagues to develop this area of expertise. These efforts brought focus to the field of children's headache.

His sensitivity to the emotional aspects of headache is legendary. His focus on depression and its treatment as a component of headache therapy was very important. Dr. Diamond was a pioneer in what is now called C.A.M. (Complementary and Alternative Medicine). His work emphasized the value of biofeedback as a therapeutic modality that could modulate pain.

His contributions to the field of headache have been recognized and acclaimed nationally and internationally. Dr. Diamond was the first recipient of the Lovshin Lectureship at the Cleveland Clinic Foundation, and served as president of the American Association for the Study of Headache, which is now called the American Headache Society. The AHS also presented the Lifetime Achievement Award to him in 1999.

His recognition that the education of patients, allied healthcare providers, and physicians could improve the lot of tens of thousands of patients was one of his major contributions. He actively worked on behalf of the patient, the public, and physicians so that headache could receive wider recognition. Dr. Diamond generously gave of his time and treasure to aid these efforts, and was a spokesperson for headache in the national media.

His organizational skills are unequaled. He personally organized postgraduate courses to spread the word about headache and improve care. These efforts were recognized locally, nationally, and internationally. His kindness and concern, always putting the welfare of his patients first, earned him the title of Mr. Headache.

This book allows readers to both understand Dr. Diamond's contributions to the field of headache and integrates his accomplishments in the history of headache as a medical specialty. His hundreds of articles, multitude of books, thousands of presentations—both lay and scientific—and numerous honors and awards cement his position in the Headache Hall of Fame.

A. David Rothner, M.D.
Chairman Emeritus of the Section of Child Neurology
Director of the Pediatric/Adolescent Headache Program
Cleveland Clinic
Cleveland, Ohio

1. You Saved My Life!

In a series of cards and letters that Dr. Seymour Diamond received after announcing his retirement from the Diamond Headache Clinic, there's a phrase that appears frequently and is most often followed by an exclamation point: "You saved my life!"

You might expect that statement in a letter to an emergency-room physician who'd literally helped his patients cheat death when they'd suffered physical trauma from automobile accidents or other violent disasters, but Seymour is a headache doctor. And these expressions of gratitude come from people who suffered from diseases that had no treatment—and little respect as an actual disease—until Dr. Diamond, with his pioneering headache-medicine mentors and peers, accepted their patients' head pain complaints as legitimate and treatable medical conditions.

"Thanks for saving my life! Until you took my case, I was on a downward spiral. You made all the difference in getting me turned around," states one letter from a man in Decatur, Illinois.

"Congratulations on all that you have accomplished to help young and old eliminate painful headaches and truly *live life again.* Thank you for giving me my life back!" says another from a woman in Chicago. She goes on to add, "I have known you for over thirty years, and I have seen your determination, passion, compassion, humility, pride, understanding, patience, and love of your work and patients. That was your success, and it continues!"

A woman from Kalamazoo, Michigan, says, "I'll never be able to express my gratitude for your being the famous doctor who *really believed* there were these awful headaches. Thousands must share in the miracles you gave us. I found hope from day one when I first saw you. You patted me on the knee and said, 'I'll help you …' After seeing nineteen doctors over a seven-year period, I knew you'd help me. Several days later, I awoke headache-free—Wow! How blessed I've been to know you as a doctor and a true friend."

A fellow M.D. from California begins her letter with that same familiar phrase, "Thank you sincerely for saving my life! Your care was exceptional, beyond mere competence. (A UCLA neurologist and a Stanford psychiatrist have been competent, but unsuccessful.) Upon regaining consciousness and clarity, I was curious to parse the elements explaining why you at the Diamond Headache Clinic succeeded so well where others had not. May I offer a few ideas?

"Your initial assessment was performed by a highest-skilled physician, not a generalist, with speed, thoroughness, precise neurological exam, in-depth history, and rapid-processing through 'rule-out' imaging.

"Diamond Headache Clinic's core is a select team of headache-dedicated experts with very extensive (half a century) clinical experience. The team is unique, well-organized, and 'on the same page.' Leadership is evident.

"The nursing team members are all fluent in treatment protocols, dosing, side effects, and outcome benchmarks. The R.N. team was confident, proud of their association with the Diamond Headache Clinic, and expressed loyalty and affection for the DHC medical faculty.

"A prominent emphasis on nonpharmacological treatment with great respect for (a) brilliant psychological evaluation, (b) salient physical therapy assessment, and (c) classical biofeedback and relaxation rehearsal made very user-friendly.

"As a migraineur for thirty-six years," she continues, "I happily report no need for a single triptan or opioid in the fifteen weeks since discharge from DHC. Diamond Headache Clinic has a master plan that is standard of care. If only DHC could clone itself!"

The traits witnessed by this thankful headache sufferer came as no accident or coincidence. In fact, Seymour has put much effort into giving his patients a premium level of care, right down to the finest details, including his greeting when he meets them for the first time. Here's an excerpt from a chapter on the history of headache clinics that Seymour wrote for Dr. Frederick G. Freitag's book *Establishing a Headache Center—From Concept to Practice*:

"I learned to greet all patients with a smile and by shaking their hands. The reason that I discuss this scenario in a chapter on the history of headache clinics is because one of the Diamond Headache Clinic's keys to success was a friendly approach to patients who had been alienated by other physicians. Headache patients are often confronted by a lack of friendliness, indifference, and misconceptions by health care professionals on the nature of headache. The patient with chronic pain, including headache, is seeking empathy as well as treatment. As a matter of rule, I always try to know something personal about the patient (job, children, hobbies), and try to establish a personal relationship. This openness may produce more insight into the patient's headaches, and facilitate the management of his or her condition. Another feature of a successful practice is to avoid long waiting times at your office, which is unacceptable and creates a barrier between you and your patient. Finally, when dealing with patients, check your ego at the door."

Seymour's methods have never been secret. In fact, he's published seventy-three books and nearly five hundred papers, alone and with coauthors, and he's delivered hundreds of speaking presentations, including thirty symposia and thirty-four special lectures.

He's appeared as a headache expert on all the major television networks (ABC, CBS, NBC, CNN, Fox) on such programs as *Today Show, Larry King Live, 48 Hours, Early Edition, ABC News with Ted Koppel, Dr. Art Ulene,* and *CBS Morning News.*

He's visited most U.S. states and a number of foreign countries, sharing his treatment knowledge along the way on meetings and discussions. In the early days of his Diamond Headache Clinic, he often invited other doctors to visit his practice to learn his methods. In the heyday of headache as a new medical specialty, the Diamond Headache Clinic reigned supreme.

"I was an energetic guy!" he laughs about it today, but it was his intelligence, education, curiosity, and that energy level, fueled by the problems presented by his patients, that drove him to research and discover new ways to help them manage their headache problems.

Seymour was instrumental in creating the first nonprofit foundation, the National Migraine Foundation, for lay people as well as physicians to benefit from current knowledge of headache treatments. He later reformed the organization into its current iteration, the National Headache Foundation, with its continued purpose to offer assistance to headache sufferers in need.

He fought battle after battle to get insurance coverage for his patients, particularly those requiring inpatient care at his affiliated hospital units, when managed care programs threatened to deny them proper treatment. Ultimately, he formed a committee that created a new standards of care document (instructions for doctors to follow in treatment) specifically for headache patients.

Seymour advised the Food and Drug Administration as a headache expert, and he fought with them over things like the drug Elavil (amitriptyline), the most prescribed drug for pain relief, that has FDA approval only as an antidepressant. When doctors prescribe a drug for anything other than its FDA approved usage, it's called "off-label" use. It's legal, and as Elavil proves, it can also be the most effective treatment.

He lists academic posts on his curriculum vitae, both past and current, including a number of professorships, instructor roles, lecturer appearances, and associate professorship positions. Sharing the knowledge has been a passion throughout his tenure as a headache specialist, and in addition to the many patients who write profusely thankful letters to their savior, a significant number of physicians owe Dr. Seymour Diamond a debt of gratitude for helping them understand the complexities of headache treatment.

Seymour will never retire completely. Today, after severing his ties with the clinic he founded, he still heads the National Headache Foundation as Executive Chairman. He's very much a hands-on individual, and at eighty-nine years of age, he still has work to do, adding to his already voluminous contribution to the welfare of headache sufferers. Born to Jewish Ukrainian/Slovakian parents who left their home countries due to religious persecution, Seymour is a member of the first American-born generation of the Diamond family. He is living proof that the American dream is attainable through hard work and determination applied intelligently. And we're lucky to have him. Except for a fortunate decision made by his parents in 1924, he might not have been born at all....

2. A Child Is Born

It was Rose Diamond's birthday. She was twenty-six years old, and she was about to enter the hospital for the birth of her second child. A brisk spring breeze off Lake Michigan tugged at her hair, and a chill rippled down her back as she looked up at the imposing face of Chicago's Michael Reese Hospital. She turned to her husband Nathan and smiled up at him, then gasped as a labor pain wracked her small figure. The baby was due.

The baby. She and Nathan had a long and difficult talk when they'd discovered her pregnancy. They had three children already, and they shared their small third-story walk-up apartment with two other adults, her mother Clara Roth and sister Esther. In 1925, only four years before the start of America's Great Depression, it was hard to earn enough money to support themselves, much less another young mouth that would need to be fed, clothed, and educated.

Nathan waited, concern etching his face, until her pain subsided, then smiled back at her, and they approached the last few steps leading to the hospital lobby.

They'd discussed "alternatives" to the birth, hesitating to use the word abortion. But they were Jewish emigrants—he from Kiev, Ukraine, and she from Kremnica, Slovakia—having come to the United States as children, and Old World family values were cherished, even here in America.

They would have the child. They would find a way to get by. They had already done more difficult things.

Nathan had left his family in Kiev at the age of twelve to escape the ire of his father's second wife, living with his grandmother until he turned eighteen. He then traveled to the United States with his cousin's family. They weren't alone.

Between 1880 and 1914, two million Jews fled the Russian Empire to escape persecution, and the exodus continued following WWI.

Repeated mob attacks, called pogroms, against Jewish citizens; the conversion of an anti-Semitic novel into a publically published document called "Protocols of the Learned Elders of Zion"; and further persecution against Jews motivated Nathan's cousin's family and thousands of others to risk the transatlantic trip to America.

They crossed the Atlantic Ocean by boat, passed through Ellis Island, and eventually made their way to Chicago, where they had relatives. Nathan found work during the day and attended English classes at night. He had a salesman's natural gift of gab, and he made a point of removing any hint of an accent, giving his new language a perfect Midwestern twang.

Rose climbed the stone steps, embraced in her husband's strong arms to assure a safe ascent. They rested a moment, then opened the hospital doors and stepped inside.

In Chicago, Nathan had met a woman, fallen in love, married, and they'd had two children, Alfred and Ann. But the marriage ultimately failed, and Nathan received custody of the children. Then, when he and Rose were married, they added daughter Idell, now eighteen months old.

Nathan was a likable man. He did well in sales, and eventually he'd open a clothing store in Chicago with a partner. The store would do well until the stock market crash of 1929, when they would file for bankruptcy and lose their business. After that, he'd sell insurance for Metropolitan Life, a vocation he'd approach with less enthusiasm than clothing sales but nonetheless provided a good living for his family.

The diminutive couple was directed to follow a nurse who helped Nathan with the paperwork, then showed him to the waiting room as another nurse led Rose away to be prepped for the delivery. She smiled happily. It was her birthday, and she was looking forward to the shared celebrations with her new child.

Rose Roth had traveled to America with her mother Clara Roth and three sisters under somewhat less dire circumstances than Nathan's. Life in Slovakia was hard. Religious intolerance combined with a poor standard of living drove many from their birth country. Following anti-Jewish riots in the early 1880s, and in reaction to the Reception Law (which put Jews on the same level of acceptance as Christians), the Slovak Clerical People's Party was formed to oppose liberalism and specifically limit Jewish influence. For the young mother traveling with four daughters, America seemed to offer the most promise for a bright future.

Nathan paced the waiting room, following in the footsteps of countless expectant fathers before him, worrying and wondering what was happening in the delivery room. Rose, now well sedated in the fashion of the times, wasn't worried about anything. She had been through the experience once before with little Idell, and although she was naturally concerned that the baby be born healthy, the birthing experience itself wasn't high on her list of concerns. As the time approached, nurses gently eased her legs into the stirrups and encouraged her to push.

Rose, like Nathan, had arrived in the United States as a youngster, passing through Ellis Island and ultimately moving on to Chicago. The 1918 influenza epidemic, which killed more people than the sixteen million who had died in WWI, captured teenaged Rose in its grip. Some patients died within hours. Others held on for several days before their lungs filled with fluid, suffocating them. Rose received appropriate treatment and survived, but a resulting viral infection had rendered her nearly deaf, and she wore hearing aids in both ears. Rose was sensitive about the hearing aids and hid them as best she could. The handicap also made her reluctant to join in her husband's business-related social gatherings due to her inability to hear the conversation clearly and reply in a comfortable manner.

But on this night, she was otherwise healthy, happy, married to a man she'd admired even when he'd been married to his first wife, and ready to give birth to their second child together.

As Rose lay exhausted, the sound of a light slap echoed through the otherwise quiet delivery room followed a split second later by a hearty yowl.

On April 15, 1925, Rose gave birth to a healthy infant whose tiny wristband read "Boy Diamond."

Two of her sisters, following Jewish tradition, had named their firstborn male children "Samuel" in memory of their deceased father. Rose felt that another Samuel would be confusing. So, she and Nathan honored their little boy with the name Schmiel Moshe, her father's Hebrew name. But the name that would become well-known in the world of headache medicine would be Seymour Diamond.

3. Times Were Different Then

"**I**'m lucky to be here," he says eighty-seven years later in his high-rise apartment overlooking Chicago's famed Lake Shore Drive and beyond it, Lake Michigan. The year is 2012.

Morning light filters in through translucent ceiling-to-floor blinds hung over huge picture windows. It reflects red-gold highlights onto the nearest wall when it strikes the collection of antique microscopes, safely ensconced in a tall glass display case. Most are made of polished brass, guided through their magnifying motion by knurled knobs and intricate gears. There's even one crafted from wood for young early nineteenth-century wannabe scientists called a Nuremberg Toy Tripod Microscope. Others date back to the 1600s.

A colorful glass bowl from the Baskets series by sculptor Dale Chihuly refracts another filtered sunbeam into a fan-shaped peacock-tail pattern across the contemporary glass-topped coffee table. A smaller multicolored glass bowl created by Lino Tagliapietra catches some of the Chihuly-enhanced beams, bouncing them onward into the room.

The back walls of the living room are lined with gray polished wood bookcases and electronic entertainment cabinets, designed by his architect/designer daughter Judi Diamond-Falk, as is the entire half-floor apartment.

Art defines the other walls. A Walt Kuhn oil painting of a nude enhances one spot, and a Ben Shahn pen-and-ink caricature of a man fills a nook. Max Weber's tiny painting "The Conversation" sits astride a miniature easel on a low bookcase among coffee-table books about other artists. Musicians sound silent strains in a painting by French-Jewish painter Mané Katz. And there's more. Much more. It's a private contemporary art gallery.

Missing are two earlier acquisitions: "Old Fisherman" by George Bellows, a 24" x 19" oil on canvas painting from the early 1900s, and "Washer Women," a smaller oil painting created by New Hope School impressionist Robert Spencer. Both were donated to Chicago's Terra Foundation for American Art as a "Gift of Seymour and Elaine Diamond."

Doormen in Seymour Diamond's high-rise building greet visitors in the porte cochere, three hundred feet below at street level as a security team watches for any cause for alarm in the newcomers' behavior, before electronically opening the heavy wooden gate that leads to the elevators. The doormen also run a pretty good football pool, in which Seymour participates with advice from his youngest daughter, journalist Amy Diamond. Somehow he wins more than she does, a fact that defies explanation.

Middle daughter, Merle, followed her dad's example and became a physician. She works in the family practice as Managing Director of the Diamond Headache Clinic, which Seymour founded in 1974.

This luxurious residence is a far cry from the pedestrian three-story walk-up where Seymour lived during his early childhood years.

The conversation pauses, waiting for the raucous clanging of the late nineteenth-century French long case clock—which signals the time with a minor cacophony of whirring gears, clacking levers, and off-key chimes—to cease. One of Seymour's daily chores is to reset the cylinder-shaped weights that power the device. He does so now, pulling downward on the chains that raise the weights.

"Times were hard, and I know my parents talked about alternatives. But I want you to know that when I was older, they explained the situation to me and expressed their regret for having ever considered it.

"It affected the way I look at abortion. I'm not pro-abortion. It might have been my only chance in this world."

He smiles slightly and shrugs. "Times were different then." It's a theme that will recur frequently throughout his long and eventful life.

Immigrants looking for homes in a new country are inclined to gather with others of their own nationality, race, or religion. Doing so allows continuation of treasured traditions, a familiar language, national pride, and a willingness to work together to find their way in a strange new country. That's just common sense, but it also creates local geographic separatism when areas are defined by their residents: an Irish neighborhood or a Spanish barrio, for example.

As the localized ethnicities vie for space, conflicts between them arise, as any urban family can verify. When a family moves into a neighborhood that doesn't match its own social characteristics, it's harder still, and the Diamond family lived in an area south of Chicago's Logan Square that was primarily occupied by former residents of Germany, Norway, and Sweden. For a Jewish kid named Seymour from an Eastern European family, conflict was inevitable.

"I had to learn to fight." he recalls. "It was a particular gang of kids. I was pretty well beaten up. My mom and dad were pretty upset by it. My mom asked my dad to go to the school and find out who they were and ask the school to take care of it." He pauses in reflection. "I survived it."

It's easy to see how a tendency toward tenaciousness would develop under such living conditions, a strength that would carry Seymour through a challenging childhood and into the worlds of medicine and business in coming years. It's a trait he treasures today and credits with much of his success.

He also learned a more positive version of tenacity from his dad's work ethic. Nathan sold insurance in a time that was far different from today. He was assigned an area to serve, which included both initial sales and then collection of premiums. The work required long hours, and he typically didn't arrive home until 7:00 or 8:00 p.m. He supplemented that income by plying his sales techniques in a Maxwell Street clothing store on the weekends. Seymour remembers his dad's dedication and feels he learned a good lesson in how to succeed simply by trying hard and never giving up.

The online Encyclopedia of Chicago describes Maxwell Street: "For about one hundred years, Maxwell Street was one of Chicago's most unconventional business—and residential—districts. About a mile long and located in the shadow of downtown skyscrapers, it was a place where businesses grew selling anything from shoestrings to expensive clothes."

The encyclopedia goes on to describe its inhabitants as immigrants from Germany, Ireland, Poland, Bohemia, and "most prominently, Jews, especially those escaping czarist Russia, Poland, and Romania.

"Goods on card tables and blankets competed with goods in sidewalk kiosks and stores. Sunday was its busiest day since the Jews worked on the Christian Sabbath, when stores were closed in other parts of the city.

"Merchants battled city officials to keep Maxwell Street alive despite its reputation for crime and residential overcrowding. Its eastern section was destroyed in the mid-1950s for the Dan Ryan Expressway. In the 1980s and 1990s, virtually all of the rest was razed for athletic fields for the University of Illinois at Chicago. What remained of the market was moved several blocks to a place with none of the flavor of the old street."

As a youth, Seymour played baseball, the all-American sport that would become a passion, particularly in following the Chicago White Sox.

"I found some friends in the neighborhood, but not many. I played some baseball. We went to an empty lot, and we'd choose sides and we'd play. I was a fair player. I wasn't great."

Greatness would come later, although not in baseball, except when the White Sox won the World Series in 2005 as Seymour turned eighty years old. Their last world championship victory had come in 1917, before he was born, eighty-eight years earlier, and he was proud and relieved that his beloved White Sox had come through with the win at least once during his lifetime! Now he expects, hopefully, for them to do it again. Every season.

Seymour remembers one of his childhood friends with sorrow. Harold (last name withheld) was one of the youngsters who befriended Seymour and gained his affection and respect in return.

"I had one friend that I associated with closely during those years. We continued to be friends even though we didn't go to the same high school."

As an adult, Harold would marry and the couple would give birth to an autistic child whom they'd ultimately place in an institution, an act that apparently was more than Harold could bear.

"He checked into a hotel room and shot himself. It's just a tragic moment. I often think of him. I met him when I was eight or nine. We were close friends. Very well read, intelligent … a nice person."

In grade school, Seymour initially experienced problems with reading, and the school advisors recommended a special reading class. Instead, he listened to his father's advice and became a solid lifelong reader without the additional help.

"If you concentrate, pull yourself together, and spend time with reading, you'll be okay," Nathan told him, and it proved to be excellent advice, requiring young Seymour to assume responsibility for the success of his own learning process.

Throughout Seymour's youth, father Nathan stood by, always ready to speak up or help out when his son needed a hand, and one of the first things he did following his son's grade school challenges was to arrange for a happier high school experience.

"My dad saw to it. Even though we didn't live in the right district, he obtained a permit for me to attend Roosevelt High School. It was in the Albany Park area, and the population of the school was about fifty-fifty with Jewish/non-Jewish students. We lived in the district called Kelvin Park, where Jewish people were a minority," Seymour recalls. "We didn't have a car at that time. I took the bus there, and it was a longer ride than to the other school. But I managed, and he encouraged me to do that. I didn't have to fight any more."

If high school were to turn things around for young Seymour, it certainly didn't happen on his first day.

"The first day of high school, my parents wanted me to be properly dressed. So they bought me a new pair of fancy knickers and a briefcase, and I went to school that way. And I guess I was a rarity like that."

Apparently knickers and a briefcase fell far from the fashion norm at Roosevelt High School in the late 1930s. As any high school student can verify, wearing the "wrong" clothes in the transitional teenage world can create a social disaster. And in Seymour's case, the embarrassment was multiplied manifold when a student article in the school newspaper pointed out his fashion faux pas to all who may have missed it in person. Decades later, he still remembers the feeling with sadness: "It wasn't a nice thing and it really bothered me."

It was also in high school that Seymour became involved with a group of students whose influence would negatively affect his life later on.

"I associated with a group who were very bright. And at the time, I thought they were much brighter than I would ever be. And I felt very inferior," he remembers. "We had lunch every day. They were all Jewish. They were the people who believed in Socialism and Communism at that time. Many of the Russian immigrants, even though they came over because of distress, believed in Socialistic and Communistic ideas. It was probably inherented from their parents."

He set out to become one of their gang, adopting their leftist beliefs and reading publications like *Friends of the USSR* and *New Republic*.

"High school was very clannish. The only club I had was this group of what I thought were superintellectuals. I've changed my mind since that time. Most of them didn't turn out very well. None of them, except perhaps one, ever achieved success in the world."

Seymour's friends and politics changed dramatically as he matured, but that brush with "un-Americanism" in high school would return to haunt him as he applied for entrance into college.

Other high school activities included music, and Seymour learned to play the clarinet. Although he's never thought of himself as a musician and didn't continue his pursuit of the instrument, he did develop a taste for classical music during his teenage years.

It was also at Roosevelt High that Seymour received praise and encouragement from an English teacher, Ms. Moser.

"I had a teacher in my junior and senior years who liked the way I wrote and really encouraged me to write. She entered me in a citywide writing contest, where I won."

Ms. Moser apparently recognized Seymour's potential, and although he wouldn't follow the path to journalism, her support and encouragement gave him a critical boost in confidence when he needed it.

4. Confidence Found

As Seymour approached high school graduation, he began to plan for college. The problem was, like many graduating students, he didn't know what he wanted to do.

"There were no guidance counselors in those days, and my parents didn't know how to advise me," he recalls.

"I applied to University of Chicago and Northwestern University in my senior year of high school. My grades were pretty mediocre in my first two years; maybe I was immature at the time. But I started to get very high grades the last two years, and I started to gain a lot of self-confidence."

The newly-minted confidence took a hit when he wasn't accepted at either school, and in his disappointment, he looked to his sister Idell for advice.

"I was very disappointed when I received the denial letters. I was very depressed personally about it, and I was talking to my sister about it, and she mentioned a couple other schools I might like. She was attending Wright Junior College, but I didn't want to go there. One of her other suggestions was the Jesuit Catholic Loyola University. I decided to give it a try. My dad went with me because I was really a discouraged kid, and I enrolled."

At the time, Seymour was seventeen years old, too young for the WWII draft for eighteen-year-olds, and as it turned out, not destined to become a soldier. In fact, it seemed that Uncle Sam and the school system were encouraging him to become a doctor.

"Because of the war conditions, Loyola had a very limited number of courses that were *not* premedical. And I had no idea whether I wanted to go into medicine or not, but it was something for me to do, so I enrolled. I was there about a year, and received almost straight-A grades, so I gained a lot of confidence in myself.

"After I finished a year, a lot of my classmates were applying to medical school. And that's after one year! They had an accelerated program because of the war. If you were in the accelerated program and you could show you had close to the amount of two years of premed, you were eligible to get into medical school. I thought about it. Why would I want to be an army private and kill people if I could be a doctor and help them?"

Once Seymour made the decision, he again applied the tenacity and determination that had been forged early in his young life.

He looked first at the University of Illinois, where the medical school campus was in Chicago. He was hoping for entry into the state system's medical school so his father would get a resident's break on tuition fees. But here his high school liberalism spoiled an otherwise stellar opportunity.

In his interview, he responded openly to their questions, and in doing so, made the mistake of mentioning his socialistic high school escapades.

"The person who interviewed me was a really conservative doctor and he turned me down just for that reason. They didn't want anybody going to that medical school who was that liberal. And I always felt bad about it because subsequently I went to another medical school, which cost my dad a lot of money. It always bothered me later on."

He also applied to the Stritch School of Medicine at Loyola University.

"Loyola Medical School, which was part of the university, at that time, had a strict non-Catholic quota. It certainly saddened and frustrated me that students with a much lower average were getting into Loyola while I and several other Jewish students did not."

His search for medical schools continued, and he finally took a look at the Chicago Medical School, even though it didn't meet current medical school requirements.

In the early 1900s, the American Medical Association formed the Council on Medical Education (CME) to establish the minimum prior education required to enter a medical school and a definition of a proper medical education to be two years of anatomy/physiology study followed by two years of training (internship) in a training hospital.

In 1908, the CME approached the Carnegie Foundation for the Advancement of Teaching. CME asked them to review the state of U.S. medical education to determine which schools met or didn't meet the CME's published standards. The foundation's president, Henry Pritchett, selected professional educator Abraham Flexner to conduct the survey.

The Flexner Report, also called Carnegie Foundation Bulletin Number Four, was researched and written by Flexner and published in 1910. When Flexner looked into medical schools, he found that many were small units run for profit by one or two local doctors whose own training in certain instances may not have been outstanding. And critically, the schools didn't meet the CME's recommended minimum standards.

While Chicago Medical School, founded in 1912, may not have met all of Flexner's standards, it did provide another overwhelmingly popular feature. The nonprofit school supported the principle that admission should be judged on merit alone. Women and minorities, who were excluded from fully-approved schools, could learn medicine there.

And it produced competent doctors.

"In order to get a license, you had to take the Illinois license exam—a very stiff exam—it wasn't like just taking your driver's test. It was a three-day, sit-down test," Seymour explains. "And in the ten years before I attended, the school's graduates were either equal or higher in these exams even though it was not an approved medical school at that time. It became an approved medical school the year after I graduated, by the way."

For young Seymour Diamond, it was a career-saving possibility, but he still had work to do. Not for the first time in his life, nor would it be the last, an opportunity presented itself, and he grasped it firmly.

"Because of the war conditions, they had certain regulations that I had to complete before I could get admitted to my first year at the Chicago Medical School. I needed about twenty-four classroom hours, which is a lot of hours, and a lot of it was very tough, like comparative anatomy ... not easy courses, like English, for example."

Currently studying at Loyola, Seymour increased his workload in an attempt to make up the needed classroom hours, but it wasn't enough.

"I could only pick up sixteen hours at Loyola. So I picked up more hours at DePaul after I finished school at Loyola. And these were rough courses that required a lot of memory. I shudder to think if I had to do the same thing today.

"Then in the evening I went to Central YMCA College, which is now Roosevelt University in Chicago. There I picked up courses like philosophy and psychology for three hours in the evening. Then I would go home and prepare for the following day's exams. I would stay up all night. I had an A-minus average when I finished and went on to medical school."

If attending three schools at once weren't enough, Seymour also kept a job selling Florsheim shoes on the weekends.

And it never got any easier. When he attended Chicago Medical School, he went from the three-schools/one-job workload to working three jobs while succeeding in a highly competitive medical school curriculum.

"I did premed in a year and a half. I was thrown into a very intelligent, studious group. Much different than college! I really had to work hard at my grades because of the competition. I completed medical school in three years."

Seymour recalls an amusing situation when he and his dad met with Dr. John J. Sheinin, Dean of the Chicago Medical School, about enrollment. Although neither Nathan nor Seymour would ever be described as tall, Dr. Sheinin's height didn't exceed five feet, and it must have bothered him.

"When we went into his office, I noticed that his desk was on a raised platform. And the place where Dad and I sat was a low, very soft couch, so that when we sat down, we sank into it and felt very small in comparison!" Seymour laughs at the memory.

Seymour speaks highly of Dr. Sheinin, although he suffered an embarrassing moment during one of the dean's lectures in which the subject was the nervous system.

"We were sitting in class and Dean Sheinin was giving a lecture. He was known to pick people out of the audience and use them as 'teaching methods.' He'd been talking about how nerves are often named after the organ they service.

"Soon enough, he points to me, asks my name, and says 'Diamond, do you know the name of the nerve that innervates the larynx?' And I really didn't. I was nervous, and I didn't know. And I hadn't studied that. So he looks at me, and he says, 'When did the War of 1812 take place?' It was a great clue, but I was so nervous, I said 'It's the 1812 Nerve?'

"You understand? [Laughing] It's the laryngeal nerve, of course, named after the organ it serves just like the 1812 War is named after the time it happened. Everybody kidded me about it for months."

Despite the increased effort required for medical school, he still needed a job. Or three.

"I worked at Florsheim Shoes on Saturdays. It paid a fairly good amount. Then after my first year in medical school, I became friendly with one of the seniors who [was] graduating, and he asked me if I wanted his job at the medical school. I would come in at noon and relieve the librarian. And when the library closed at 5:00 p.m., it was my job to wash down the floors. It was also open two nights from 5:00 to 7:00 p.m. I would sit and study, as well as help any students who might be utilizing the library. It was a good opportunity. I learned about books, I learned about journals, what's relevant about reading to be a good doctor. I also got another job for three nights a week besides that, working as an extern. They usually hired medical students to do histories on patients at the hospitals, so I was working three jobs. I was an energetic person."

It was the extern job that captured Seymour's imagination, however, and cemented his decision about becoming a doctor.

"I had a chance to work with the residents at Franklin Boulevard Hospital who were learning surgery. A big surgical group owned it. I could scrub in and watch surgeries and see a lot of pathology. It was a wonderful experience while going to school. It really invigorated me about medicine."

With a schedule like that, it's a wonder that Seymour had time for anything resembling a social life.

"I had dated some nurses from the hospital, but I never dated anybody who was of my heritage. I'd gone out with girls superficially, but never anything serious. My parents weren't worried about me getting married before I finished school because none of the girls I brought home were Jewish."

But all that was about to change. It happened when a doctor at Franklin Boulevard made a simple suggestion.

"One of the resident's names was Phillip Lerner. He was a surgical resident. And he was a very nice man, much older than I, and he kept telling me he had two nice nieces that I should date. And Elaine was one of them. I called her up, and we had our first date."

Little did he know that he was about to meet the brilliant young woman who would become his life partner.

5. Elaine

"So my uncle went up to Seymour and said, 'Please call one of these girls; their mothers are driving me crazy!'" The former Elaine Flamm, now Elaine Diamond for the past sixty-three years, smiles at the memory. She had recently broken an engagement with another suitor, and apparently her mother was anxious to make up for lost time.

"That was college time," she muses. "There were young interns and externs, and my mother's older sister and my mother were both after my uncle to have one of the young doctors call us. They felt that marrying a doctor would be a very good thing."

Seymour did indeed call Elaine, and he asked her out on a date. Here each of them individually recalls an evening that sounds like a scene from a romantic comedy.

She: "I remember our first date vividly because it poured! We went down to Rush Street to a nice Italian restaurant, and we talked."

He: "I took her to an Italian restaurant on Rush Street. And she didn't eat a lot, which was good. I was afraid—I didn't have a lot of money then!"

She: "And then we walked home along the beach in the park; in those days you could do it. It was a nice night, but then it started to rain, and so we hung out near a park restroom shelter and talked. And talked. And talked!"

He: "And then a thunderstorm, a tremendous thunderstorm occurred. We were in the park, and I was very cognizant of the fact that lightning could hit us very easily in those circumstances.

The shelter was in the park just off the Outer Drive, and we ran to it. We were there for almost an hour, talking some more."

She: "Eventually we decided that, well, we were just going to have to get wet; it didn't stop raining. And so he went out and found a cab. And that was the first date."

He: "As the rain eased, we were both drenched as well. I flagged down a cab on Lake Shore Drive while Elaine waited in the shelter—he stopped on the Drive, which they're not supposed to do—and picked us up. I took her home and then paid the cab because I couldn't afford for him to take me home. I walked from there about a half mile to catch a streetcar home."

Popular Diamond family myth has Elaine arriving home from the date and announcing to her mother that Seymour was the man she was going to marry. "Actually," she says today, "I said I'd either marry Sey or someone just like him. We really hit it off!"

Not long thereafter, Seymour gave her his class ring. It signified their engagement, although over the next few years she'd switch it "from left hand to right hand and then back again and then back again!"

"He was young," she recalls, "and his parents weren't eager for him to make any firm commitments at that time."

Then she adds, "Finally my dad said, 'One way or the other, figure it out.' He was a very quiet man, but he was a very smart man in so many ways. He was the one who told me, when I was engaged to this other person, that it was all right to end that engagement. He cleared the way. I guess he cleared the way for Seymour to make a decision."

She laughs. "This was early times! Early, early times!" Issues that seem earth-shattering or life-changing when one is young often provide humorous recollections later in life.

Elaine's family had settled in the United States earlier than Seymour's. It was her father's generation that became the first born in the United States, her grandfather having emigrated from Poland, her grandmother from Russia.

Persecution of Polish Jews dates back to the thirteenth century following two hundred years of acceptance. Early settlers were part of a migration from Western Europe to Poland, where they were welcomed under the rule of Boleslaus III in the eleventh century. His interest was in developing the economic structure of his country, a plan that succeeded, for Jewish merchants soon formed the core of the Polish economy.

A combination of the Roman Catholic Church and nearby German states did their best to change matters despite the laws made by the Polish government to protect Jews into the 1300s. But through the centuries, disfavor and violence against Jews increased, influenced by religious competition and the invading Russians.

In the years Elaine's father's family finally left Poland—the late nineteenth century—pogroms (mob violence against Jews) had continued. Like Russian emigrants, including her mother's family, Elaine's father's family chose to leave Poland behind and make the transatlantic trip to America. And once here, they prospered!

Her only memory of her paternal grandfather is "someone in black sitting at what I think was a dining room table holding a book, a Torah, I think." It's the memory of a very young child. She never knew her paternal grandmother, who apparently died at a young age. Elaine adds, "So, the kids basically raised themselves. It was a nice family; they supported each other."

Elaine's father, Samuel Flamm, was the second oldest of seven children, her uncle Irving being the eldest. Irving became a lawyer, and her dad was a retailer, first selling linoleum and paint, later opening a grocery store.

Elaine's mother, originally called Bessie Melamed, was one of five children who passed through Ellis Island en route to Chicago. "Melamed" means "teacher" in Hebrew. An older sister married a man with the last name of Lerner, and although the full story is unknown, his presence influenced the entire family to change their names to Lerner, as well.

Her closely-knit family experienced American-style culture shock when an aunt married a man from Mississippi. The aunt desperately wanted family down there, so to support his sister, Elaine's dad sold his paint and linoleum store, and the family moved. After living an urban life among others with similar backgrounds in the North, life in the American South was "interesting." They lasted six months before Elaine's mother insisted they return to her beloved Chicago and family.

Elaine's childhood experiences in Mississippi included Christian prayers recited every morning in school, restrooms, drinking fountains, even grocery stores marked "White Only" and public parks with "Negro Areas." They were a successful family, thanks to Samuel's retail sales skills, and there were good business opportunities there. "We lived very nicely because there was lots of help for very little money, but it was a whole different way of life." She refers to Kathryn Stockett's book, *The Help*, saying that its telling of incidents related to the racist Jim Crow Laws closely reflects the reality of her life there, quite a shock for a Northern-born Chicago woman.

Back in Chicago, Elaine attended college at the University of Chicago, earning a degree in social work as Seymour continued his work in medical school. As graduation drew near, so did marriage.

6. Medical School and Marriage

Seymour's life flowed inexorably onward, ever busy with his medical school studies, his three jobs, and his romance with Elaine. "I had a lot of stamina in those days," he laughs.

"I liked her, she liked me, and we went out many times after that." The pair dated for six or eight weeks before Seymour introduced her to his parents. Being the first Jewish girl young Seymour had brought home caused his parents some concern, fearing perhaps that his studies would suffer while his marriage prospects would grow stronger. In those days, Jews didn't marry outside their ethnicity as a matter of appropriate behavior; in earlier times, they'd have been severely ostracized. But Seymour's parents needn't have worried; Seymour was focused on completing all of his endeavors successfully.

His intensity and sense of purpose are reflected decades later in the disappointment and disbelief he expresses in a story about a fellow medical school student.

"We worked with a cadaver in anatomy courses. Four of us were assigned to each cadaver because to dissect all the nerves and everything is a lot of work, a lot of time and effort. It's a good learning experience because you learn anatomy—the body—very thoroughly. And it's always in your mind after you finish that.

"The school selected the student partners by alphabet. My name is Diamond and my partner's name was Diller. And at the other side of the table were two more guys. One named Feldman, who was a friend of mine, and one named Feinstein, a med school acquaintance.

"My partner, Diller, was a nonentity! He never showed up for class; he never helped in the dissections. He was interested in music. We had practical exams where we pointed out different things on the human body, and then we took written tests. He would borrow notes from other students and actually received tremendous grades even though he didn't participate.

"Then later, when we were three months away from graduation, he quit medical school." Seymour shakes his head in disbelief as he delivers the punch line: "It turned out he was just dodging the draft!"

In their sophomore year, students would go through—as Seymour describes it, "a gigantic book ... at least ten thousand pages"—the entirety of *Cecil Medicine* under the guidance of an instructor, page by page. *Goldman's Cecil Medicine*, originally published in 1927, was "the granddaddy of general internal medicine texts ... solidly written and effectively illustrated ... and a comprehensive resource on diseases of adults," a *Journal of the American Medical Association* (JAMA) review said of the twentieth edition.

After reviewing the tome, students had been exposed, however briefly, to almost any disease that can possibly harm a human being. The trick was being able to recall them at the appropriate time, a skill shared and proven by Seymour and his best friend in medical school, Joe Goldberg.

Seymour and Joe were working in a dermatological clinic during their third year of medical school. An elderly African American man was their patient, and he complained of a band around his little toe that was constricting it, almost to the point of making it gangrenous.

"I looked at Joe, and he looked at me, and we both said, 'ainhum!' That's the disease, and it's the smallest paragraph in *Cecil Medicine*. The professor of dermatology congratulated us on our diagnosis and wrote up the case because it was that rare." Seymour and Joe were two proud and happy medical students after that evidence of their learned skills.

The word "ainhum" comes from the tribe first reported to suffer the disease in the Bahia state of Brazil, the Nagos. In their language it means "to saw," referring to the painful loss of the fifth (little) toe by (in medical terms) bilateral spontaneous amputation. (It falls off.) The word origin is thought to be African since the Nagos came to

South America through the slave trade and are related to a Nigerian tribe. In the United States, it's rare and little known.

In another incident, Seymour wasn't so happy with his pal: "He was a smooth talker and had many girlfriends among the nurses at County Hospital. He fixed me up with some of them, which was nice. When Elaine and I became informally engaged, I introduced him to Elaine. And the S.O.B. called her afterwards—he was that charming—to see if she would go out with him!" (Of course, she didn't.)

One of the least popular experiences among most students was their stint outside Chicago at the Oak Forest Infirmary. Located in the tiny village of Oak Forest, the infirmary was accessible for students who didn't own cars by riding the Rock Island Railroad, and once there, the young medical students had almost nothing to do except study.

"I would go for the week," Seymour says. "There were the rich kids who had their cars and did what they wanted to do, but there was nothing to do there. Those were the years before television. There was maybe a tavern or two, but that was about it!"

The infirmary, now called Oak Forest Hospital, is located twenty miles south of the Chicago Loop. It gave Seymour valuable medical school experience in working with patients who needed chronic care, and as he puts it, "It was a neurological treasury."

The facility had been established in 1910 as a poor farm when overcrowded conditions at the County Poor Farm in Dunning became extreme. Nearly two thousand unfortunate individuals who were destitute due to poverty, alcoholism, or mental illness lived there then, working the farmland that surrounded it and receiving care. By the early 1930s, the population had doubled and included tuberculosis sufferers as well. When Seymour did his Oak Forest stint in medical school, he estimated the population at four to five thousand patients.

"There were no home health care services then," he explains. "Patients with severe Parkinson's, central nervous system syphilis, muscular dystrophy, and others who needed chronic care had no place else to go. It was sad for them, but it provided a wonderful learning experience."

It was also an opportunity to learn from the best, because although full-time resident physicians maintained a standard daily routine, specialists were brought in to deal with the more difficult or unusual cases.

Dr. Harry Garner and Dr. Paul Woska served as professors at the Chicago Medical School, and they made the trip to Oak Forest to review the problem cases with their students.

"And that was a really great thing because we'd go over the cases, the actual cases, and they would talk about the treatments and the diseases themselves," Seymour recalls.

"Paul Woska gave his lectures early in the morning at 7:00 or 8:00 a.m., and if you missed them, he would think nothing of flunking you. He was strict about attendance taking. He wanted everybody there, and he did one of his lectures early on Monday morning! It didn't bother me because I took the train out the night before.

"But one of the seniors missed the local train. There was a later train that went on all the way to California, but that train didn't stop at Oak Forest. He was an older guy, about thirty-eight, and he looked distinguished, tall, and he carried a medical bag with his instruments in it. And he was nearly hysterical because he knew Dr. Woska was going to flunk him!

"So he took the California express train and told the conductor that he was a doctor, that he was scheduled for surgery, and that it was critical that the engineer halt at Oak Forest to let him off. So, the train made an unscheduled stop, which allowed him to attend Dr. Woska's lecture.

"It all went well until a few days later when the railroad called the infirmary to see how the surgery had gone!" Seymour adds with a chuckle. The school did not see the humor in the story nor did they reward the student's creativity or persistence. He did receive a failing grade, and he did have to repeat his senior year.

Already carrying a heavy burden of classes and part-time work, Seymour added to his busy schedule by volunteering to co-edit a scientific journal published by the school and its students, *The Chicago Medical School Quarterly*, no doubt drawing on the encouragement and success he'd enjoyed in Ms. Moser's high school English class.

He also got to work determining where he'd serve his internship. Graduation would provide his Bachelor of Medicine degree, but during those years, an aspiring young doctor had to complete a year of internship working with full-fledged physicians in a student hospital setting to qualify for a Doctor of Medicine license.

Since the Chicago Medical School was not one of the Flexner-approved schools, Seymour's search was more difficult.

"I sent out various applications, got rejections, and finally was accepted at the University of Arkansas Medical Hospital in Little Rock. Now this was a real coup because it was a teaching hospital. I told my friends about it, and eventually three of us were accepted there."

As medical school drew to an end, wedding bells filled the air, and they set the date for June 20, 1948.

Graduation and wedding ceremonies nearly collided when the school rescheduled the graduation at the last minute, placing it just one day before the wedding. Based on Seymour's energetic activity level with school, three jobs, and a girlfriend, it probably seemed normal to him to graduate one day and get married the next.

Friends and family gathered at the Webster Hotel on Lincoln Park West for a traditional Jewish wedding ceremony. The upscale lakefront hotel, one of many designed by Gustav H. Gottschalk, had hosted individuals both famous and infamous over its lifetime. Eleanor Roosevelt had stayed there, as had Al Capone. It was also the scene of a famous jazz recording session where Jelly Roll Morton and the Red Hot Peppers performed for RCA's microphones.

But on this happy day, the venue's primary guests were Seymour, clad in a tuxedo, and Elaine, radiant in her white wedding dress. Elaine's sister Barbara joined the wedding party as a bridesmaid; Seymour's best man was his childhood friend Harold, the friend who would later commit suicide.

The honeymoon may have given Elaine a sobering sample of what life would be like living with her brand-new doctor husband: "We didn't have any money to go anywhere, so we stayed at a hotel on the north side of Chicago for a couple of days."

And what did they do for fun? Elaine laughs, "There was an AMA (American Medical Association) convention in town, so we went to the convention. We were doing medical stuff from day one!"

She was now twenty-one years old, and Seymour was twenty-three. His internship in Little Rock, Arkansas, was slated to begin on July 1—less than a week away. It was time to move!

7. Southern Living

Elaine's parents, Samuel and Bessie Flamm, supported their newlywed daughter and her husband by driving them to Little Rock and staying to help out until the young couple was settled. Seymour and Elaine packed their belongings into the Flamm's 1947 Studebaker and headed south for Arkansas, leaving Chicago behind.

In those days, apartments weren't plentiful, so the Diamonds rented a small house. Elaine had not yet found work, and Seymour earned only $25 a month for his internship position.

"We found a house for rent, but the rent was too much for one couple. It was a two-bedroom bungalow, and it had transportation nearby, so I could get to the hospital. So I talked to one of the people who came down with me, Sherman Feinstein, one of the other students. He and his wife decided to share the house with us."

As with any move to a new location, there were issues to be dealt with, differences to be sorted out.

"There were no delicatessens in Little Rock. So Elaine and I once took a two-hour bus ride back and forth to Hot Springs just to get a corned beef sandwich!" Seymour recalls.

"Little Rock had a very small Jewish population. And we attempted to go to one of the temples there one night, but people weren't welcoming. We settled there, and I went on to my internship." Seymour recalls.

"I really enjoyed it. The three of us from Chicago Medical School ran rings around the other thirty or so interns. We were sharp!

"There were some experiences we had there that I still recall … it was being there in the South when there were two drinking fountains, two toilets, the back of the bus, you know. It was a different lifestyle for two people from the Midwest. We just couldn't believe it. There were two blood banks!

"I'm going to talk about some of the things that went on there. I don't know if it's book-appropriate, but anyway … I was on Emergency Room service for the first month of my internship. And that was fun! Some days we'd see as many as one hundred to 125 people. They had no other source for care.

"I really enjoyed Emergency Room service because I saw a lot of people and helped a lot of people. One of the interesting things was Friday night in the emergency room. That's payroll night, and there was a lot of drinking. I don't think there were any drugs at that time, but a lot of drinking. And a lot of slashing. One night I counted the number of sutures I put in, in a night's service there. It was close to 450!"

As Seymour sutured his way through ER service, Elaine went job hunting.

"I had a regular bachelor's degree, and I was one year into my social work degree," she recalls. "All I needed was some field work. My folks were going to pay for my extra year. When I applied to the University of Arkansas, they didn't like my University of Chicago degree because it was a two-year degree. They weren't going to accept my early credits, and I wasn't going to start over again, so I went looking for a job.

"There were no social work jobs. Not a lot of private agencies there. So I then applied to the Department of Education, and I was suddenly teaching fifth grade without a teaching credit to my name! I was two days ahead of the kids in the curriculum," she jokes.

Her life teaching school wasn't without its rare moments. Teachers were required to teach evolution in the fifth grade.

"I was dutifully teaching it," Elaine smiles, "when a boy in worn bib overalls stood up and said, 'My pappy don't believe in that!'"

"That stopped me for moment before I tactfully replied, 'Your pappy has a right to his opinion, and we'll respect that right.'"

Teaching wasn't for Elaine as a full-time career ("I did NOT like teaching. Maybe if I'd been prepared … but anyway, it paid, and with his $25 a month, we got by."). But she soldiered on as Seymour kept busy at the university hospital. By now he'd moved on from Emergency Room duty to the Contagious Diseases sector.

"That was probably one of the most fascinating services I've ever experienced. I'd read about a lot of these diseases, but I never expected to ever see some of them! I saw Rocky Mountain spotted fever, tularemia, ailments that you wouldn't see even at Cook County in Chicago. These were rare, contagious diseases!

"Those were also the years of the big polio epidemic. We were so busy with the polio patients that the ward was overflowing. We had them in the halls, all over, because we couldn't take care of all of them. We didn't have the room. And actually you didn't want to put them in another part of the hospital.

"They would bring somebody in, and naturally they had the symptoms of polio: stiff neck and running a high fever. Nowadays if I were to see a case like that, I would do a spinal tap and send it out to the laboratory to get an immediate reading. But during those days, we did our own lab work. We would look at the spinal fluid and make the diagnosis before sending it along to the laboratory for confirmation.

"There were two cases that were really interesting. One: a mother came in with a four-year-old boy who had the symptoms—stiff neck, fever—and still breastfeeding! I examined the child, and I did the spinal tap. When I got the results, I went out and told the mother, 'Your child has polio, and we're going have to keep him here.'"

The woman didn't want to leave her son (possibly thinking he'd starve without her to feed him), but there was no room for her to stay overnight.

"We had no room for any parents. We were in the middle of an epidemic and all the beds were filled, so I told her she couldn't stay. Then she reached down into the cotton dress she was wearing and pulled out a pistol!

"'I'm a-stayin'!' she said.

"'Yes, you are,' I replied. We arranged sleeping arrangements even though the contagious ward was markedly overpopulated, and she was happy we did it."

The other case Seymour felt was interesting involved tularemia, also called rabbit fever or deer fly fever. It's often spread through ticks and deer flies and typically presents itself as lesions on the hands. People who own and handle domestic rabbits are susceptible. It's very rare that the disease infects other parts of the body, but it does happen.

"The patient, an adult male, came in with pneumonia, but it looked very queer on the X-ray. It wasn't a normal pneumonia. We cultured his sputum, and it turned out that it was a very rare case of tularemic pneumonia.

"I went to the library and looked up 'tularemic pneumonia.' It was almost always fatal because you couldn't isolate it. It was in the lungs, so eventually, the patient couldn't breathe anymore and died.

"I was an avid reader of medicine and all its literature at the time. My library days in medical school certainly paid off. I knew that penicillin was about to come into use—it was being used on the troops, and we would be able to get it—but penicillin didn't work on this type of infection.

"There are gram-positive and gram-negative bacteria that cause infections. Penicillin had already been discovered and was very effective in gram-positive infections. There was only early research on antibiotics for gram-negative infections. This one was gram-negative. I had seen in one of the journals that a man by the name of Waksman had developed a drug called streptomycin. It was purely in experimental stages. So, with permission of the authorities there at the hospital, we contacted him. He sent some to the hospital to try on our patient. And he got better!"

Selman Waksman, Ph.D., was a microbiologist and biochemist who coined the word *antibiotic* during his study of organisms that live in the soil and their decomposition. He discovered more than twenty antibiotics, including streptomycin, for which he received the 1952 Nobel Prize in Physiology or Medicine. Streptomycin was the first effective treatment for tuberculosis.

In a groundbreaking case such as Seymour's tularemic pneumonia patient, doctors like to keep records, write papers, and actively share their findings with the rest of the world. In this instance, Seymour wanted his patient to stay in the hospital for a series of X-rays to show the progression of the recovery. Unfortunately, the patient didn't want to stay.

"He was from the hill country, and if we'd let him out, we'd never see him again," Seymour recounts. "We kept him until he ran away one day! We came in the next morning, and he wasn't there!" And as Seymour feared, the healed patient was never heard from again.

Young Dr. Diamond was quickly building experience that would serve him well in coming years. Tending to everyday diseases is rewarding and provides a good living, but treating patients who have challenging medical problems with cutting-edge knowledge and medicines was to become Dr. Seymour Diamond's professional lifestyle.

But it wasn't to last, at least not at the University of Arkansas Medical Hospital.

"Four or five months into the internship, I was called down to the office of the president of the university. When I arrived, my two other friends from Chicago Medical School were already there. There were four of the professors there, and they said that when they accepted us, they didn't know we came from an unapproved school. And they wanted us to resign. I didn't know from lawyers or stupidity, and we all resigned. We should have sought the counsel of our dean at the Chicago Medical School, Dr. Sheinin.

"Apparently, one of the interns there with me—and I still know him very well—kept bragging to the other residents that we were so good even though we came from an unapproved school. Other interns hearing this went to the administration."

Seymour found himself out of his internship and out of work. Fortunately, when he was working on the polio ward, the state health department oversaw the work, and he became familiar with one of the administrators.

"He heard about my misfortune, so he called and asked me if I would like to work for him at the health department. He gave me a job as a consultant.

"During those years, there were many army camps around, and syphilis and gonorrhea were rampant. I worked administering tests, and it was interesting. We would go into small towns and stay in local hotels. We had a truck with loud speakers that we would drive around announcing, 'Do you have bad blood?' (We didn't use the word syphilis.) Or, 'Do you have a discharge?' (Rather than say gonorrhea.) We used those terms because the population wasn't educated in venereal diseases. And we set up a tent or a facility—it depended on how big the town was—and asked people to come in and be tested.

"It was a fascinating experience in my life! They were trying to strike out venereal diseases. Gonorrhea was prevalent then and is rampant again right now, especially among our young gay population, but you rarely see syphilis anymore. And it had such a high morbidity with paralysis, dementia, and heart manifestation.

"But it was also a period where we trying to prevent this morbidity, to catch the disease early. You could diagnose syphilis by a blood test, while you could determine gonorrhea by looking at the smear of the discharge. And I did this for about six months.

"Funny story: I was working about 240 miles from Little Rock in Fort Smith. I had a government car, which was great because the war had forced gas rationing, but I was on a government expense account. I got a call one morning from the office in Little Rock, not from my friend who got me the job, but from his superior. He said, 'Seymour, I want you to come up and see me tonight.' And I said, 'Can I wait until I come back there in two days?' He said, 'No. I want to see you tonight.'

"So I drove all the way to Little Rock and went to his house. And he said to me, 'Seymour, do you like working for the health department?' And I said, 'Yes, of course I do.' And he said 'Well, you sort of embarrassed everybody with your expense account. We would like to have you continue working, but can I show you how you should do an expense account?' And he showed me how to do an expense account. And I continued to have the job. His complaint? I wasn't spending enough money; I was too cheap!"

Even while Seymour was working for the health department in Arkansas, he and Elaine continued to search for a new internship opportunity.

"Elaine and I would write letters. There's a list of all the approved hospitals in the United States. There are thousands and thousands of them. We filled out application after application."

Seymour had worked for the health department for about six months when he received an important phone call.

"I got a call from one of my Chicago Medical School classmates, the one who'd talked too much and caused us to lose our University of Arkansas Hospital internships. He'd gotten an internship in Columbus, Ohio, at a large hospital. It was a large Methodist facility known as White Cross Hospital. It had eight hundred beds—a large hospital! It was a teaching hospital connected with the Ohio State University (OSU), which was a great thing. He thought I should call them and apply, and I did. I was accepted, and Elaine and I moved to Columbus, Ohio."

8. Seymour Goes Neural

Once again, Seymour's in-laws, Samuel and Bessie Flamm, helped out with the move. Seymour and Elaine packed their meager belongings into the Studebaker and struck out for Columbus, Ohio, to face the next challenges of their young lives.

White Cross Hospital began life as Protestant Hospital in 1891. The name was changed to White Cross in 1922. The name would change again in 1961, and today it's known as Riverside Methodist Hospital. Among its claims to fame is that it "leads the field of neurosciences with one of the largest neurology and stroke programs in the U.S. with innovative treatments offered for brain and stroke," according to the hospital's website. Here, Seymour would begin his life's adventure in neurology.

But first they needed a place to live. As in Little Rock, apartments were scarce, and they wound up living in the Neal House Hotel, a huge, red-brick building located just across from the state capitol.

By today's standards, the rates seem extremely low, but in 1949's economy, the $8 per night fee for two guests ($6 for a single) was a challenge despite Seymour's raise from $25 per month in Little Rock to $50 per month for his internship in Columbus. Seymour's schedule dictated that he work at the hospital every other night. That meant that only one person would be in the room, so on those nights, he would check out, pay the $6 rate for Elaine alone, saving $2 each time, and then check in again on the following night. On a monthly basis, that amounted to a savings of about $30, which looked good beside his $50 internship salary.

Eventually, they would find housing. Elaine explains: "We had trouble finding housing because there weren't a lot of apartments and we couldn't afford very much. But we finally found a place with a very nice woman who was a Christian Scientist."

Interestingly, their new landlord didn't believe in locking doors, and in fact, the doors on their apartment had no locks. It was an unusual and unsettling situation for the Chicago-born couple. And Elaine's dad felt the same.

"My parents visited, and although my dad wasn't a handyman, he went out, bought locks, and installed them! I was very impressed; I'd never seen my father do anything like that. But he knew Seymour worked every other night, leaving me alone in the place, so he took care of it," Elaine says, smiling at the memory.

"I loved Columbus!" she says. "I took an exam for social service to work in the field, and I got the job." She begins to say, "I got a very good score … " before humility takes over and she changes the sentence to, "I'm a good test-taker."

She continues, "I loved working in the field! We made some good friends there. We almost thought we'd stay but, you know … eventually we'd come back to Chicago."

Seymour, obviously proud, states it slightly differently: "She had the first or second best exam score in the state! She's a smart lady." He pauses a second, then adds with a sly grin, "She married me, you know?"

"She had a good job, one she liked. I was making $50 a month rather than $25 a month. But Elaine was still the bread winner," he concludes.

Elaine adds, "The early years were really kind of fun. We were just one step ahead of the paycheck, but it was all right; it worked fine. There were a lot of people in our position."

At the hospital, Seymour was thrilled by the opportunities that were presented to him.

"I had a chance to scrub in with a famous doctor whose name is on a syndrome: Dr. Robert Zollinger. It's called the Zollinger-Ellison syndrome. This was big-time for me," he reminisces.

Zollinger-Ellison syndrome is a complex condition when one or more tumors form in the pancreas, duodenum (upper intestine), or lymph nodes adjacent to the pancreas. The tumors produce the hormone gastrin that causes excessive acid to be formed in the stomach, and the result is stomach ulcers.

"Dr. Zollinger was the head of surgery at Ohio State University's College of Medicine and at White Cross, where the neurosurgical group was the largest such group in the state.

"I took a special liking to the neurosurgical service there. I always liked neurology. I'd had a close relationship with Harry Garner, who was head of the Department of Neurology at the Chicago Medical School. I liked working up the patients that came in on this service, doing their histories and doing neurological exams on them."

Dr. Robert M. Zollinger, according to his biography on the Ohio State University website, was "respected by his peers, feared by his students, and loved by his patients." He was encouraged throughout his youth by supportive parents who had complete confidence in Robert and his brother Richard, instilling in them a strong sense of self-confidence.

He began his nearly thirty-year service at Ohio State University as the chairman of the Department of Surgery in 1947. He is described as "a difficult taskmaster who expected nothing less than perfection from himself and his colleagues." A story persists that while on rounds, he was known to have fired a resident during a trip up the elevator only to rehire him by the time they had reached their destination floor.

Again from the OSU website, when Dr. Zollinger was once asked how he would like to be remembered, he responded, "They should write on my tombstone: 'teacher, surgeon, soldier, and farmer.' And my wife may remember that she says I'm an amusing fellow to live with."

In addition to Dr. Zollinger, Seymour also had the honor of working with the Neurological Associates team of Dr. Harry E. LeFever and Dr. Roy J. Secrest.

Dr. LeFever was a pioneer in neurosurgery. He'd received his medical degree in 1925, the year Seymour was born, and then studied with Dr. Harvey Cushing in Boston and with Dr. Thierry de Martel and Dr. Clovis Vincent in France. LeFever returned to Ohio in 1932, became founder/mentor for neurosurgery at Ohio State University. He was determined to establish himself as a specialist in neurosurgery despite predictions from his father, a family practice physician, that he would starve if he limited himself to brain surgery.

Fortunately, his dad was wrong, and by 1937, Dr. LeFever was well established as a neurosurgeon at White Cross Hospital. He volunteered for military service in the navy when WWII broke out, then returned to Ohio State after his military discharge. There, according to a passage on Ohio State University's website, he "immediately locked horns with the new chief of Surgery, Dr. Robert M. Zollinger."

From Seymour's perspective, it was like walking among the neurological gods. Referring to Drs. LeFever and Secrest, he recalls, "I was able to scrub in with them for long surgical procedures. Any neurosurgery at that time took from four to ten hours."

In a more mundane moment that suddenly turned exciting, Seymour was working as an intern in the general surgery area and called upon to remove the stitches from a patient's arm. The patient had broken the limb and was lying there with the arm in traction.

"It took place in a large ward, one with six people in it. I took out the stitches as gently as I could. I told him what I was doing, as I always did, and I completed the procedure. But as I walked out of the room, I instinctively felt something coming towards me, so I ducked. It was an orthopedic weight, and it hit a patient two beds away. You can imagine the force it was thrown with … it fractured the patient's skull!

"The man I'd helped was a paranoid schizophrenic, and he thought I was Jesus Christ. This is true! They called the hospital psychiatrist, who had been his psychiatrist before (whoever the psychiatrist was, he abdicated his duty). He should have had the patient hospitalized in a psychiatric institution for the criminally insane.

"But they put his arm in a cast and discharged him, which was the wrong thing to do. About a week or two went by, and Elaine started to receive calls from him, asking when I would be home. I talked to the president of the hospital staff, and he said, 'Maybe you should take a vacation with your wife for two weeks, back to Chicago.' And they would call me when I should come back. There were no provisions for that in those days, for time off. They eventually incarcerated this man with the criminally insane."

Even his in-surgery experience with the Neurological Associates team had its curious quirks.

"Neurosurgery is very precise work and can be very frustrating for both the surgeon and his assistants. The first time I scrubbed on a brain tumor operation with Dr. LeFever and Dr. Secrest, which took eight hours, I constantly heard the words, 'Damn you, Joe!' and then similar profanity at 'Joe.' They had agreed that Joe would be the person they'd cuss so they'd never get mad at each other during surgery. It took me a while to figure out that Joe was simply an anonymous recipient of the curses.

"I decided that I would like to go into neurosurgery then," Seymour adds.

But it wasn't quite that easy.

"In those days you couldn't go directly into neurosurgery," he explains. "The prerequisite was that you needed a year of general surgery. At White Cross Hospital, the residencies in surgery were filled. But they called one of their former residents and found me a position in the general surgery hospital in Cincinnati."

Once again, they piled their belongings into the Flamm's Studebaker, this time heading southwest to Cincinnati and the now defunct St. Mary's Hospital.

And again, Elaine left her social field work behind and went job hunting in Cincinnati.

"I got a job at The Jewish Hospital," she recalls, "and it was one of the best jobs I ever had. They were doing a geriatric social service program there. It was very innovative. Nobody else was doing that kind of thing. Nobody paid a lot of attention to old people."

St. Mary's Hospital, where Seymour would work, was originally founded in the mid-1800s by the Sisters of the Poor of St. Francis who moved to Cincinnati from Aix-la-Chapelle, France. It is no longer in existence today.

"One of the reasons I went there," Seymour says, "is that the head of neurology there was a former resident of the Neurological Associates group I worked with in Columbus, Dr. Robert Schlemmer. He was really nice to me and wanted me to scrub on all his neurosurgical procedures.

"However, I also became disenchanted with surgery, especially neurosurgery. Not the part about working with the patients (neurology), but with the mechanical nature of it. I didn't think I was utilizing my mind in the way I should with surgery. And I decided this was not the way I wanted to spend my life. It's one of the most important decisions I ever made ... I decided neurosurgery was just not my bag.

"Basically, there were no controls over surgeons and the procedures they do, as there are today. Dr. Schlemmer heard about a procedure they were doing in Germany for retarded children, and he spent some time over there studying it before he brought it back to the U.S.

"Now, first of all, when anyone has a retarded child, or a child with any difficulty, there is a tremendous guilty feeling in the parent. If you have anything wrong with your child, you will go out of your way, both financially and time-wise, to try to help your child. Parents will agree to almost anything they believe will help.

"So, although it wasn't an accepted procedure, and I knew of only one other institution that was also doing it, he would take children who were maybe in a 50–70 I.Q. range, and he would tie off the jugular vein. The theory for tying the vein was that more blood would stay in the brain and improve their condition.

"They claimed it helped, and some children were better after the procedure. But my explanation for the improvement is that all of a sudden, people were *trying* to teach one of these children something.

"I felt they were taking advantage of the parents' concern and guilt. I'm a pretty straight thinker, and I couldn't see any logic to it."

Other neurosurgical and psychosurgical procedures of the day added to Seymour's distaste for the specialty. One of the most dramatic procedures shares a pair of names that would give pause even to the most naive medical layperson today: "ice pick procedure" and "lobotomy."

The practice, begun in Europe in the mid 1930s, was embraced and enhanced by American neurosurgeons Walter Freeman and James W. Watts. They created a standard prefrontal procedure and called it "lobotomy." After WWII, Freeman discontinued his association with Watts, refined his procedure, and renamed it "transorbital lobotomy." That's where the ice pick comes in, as Seymour describes the procedure.

"While I was on Dr. LeFever's neurosurgical service, they did a new and controversial surgery known as transorbital leucotomy, or lobotomy. It was used for people with incurable mental disease and incurable depression.

"In this procedure, they would first electric shock a patient. Once the seizure phase of the treatment caused by the electric shock was completed, the patient was relatively unconscious. They then took an instrument modeled after a standard ice pick and poked it in through the eye socket to cut the connections to the prefrontal cortex. It was in vogue at the time, but there were no studies on it. I saw one patient die and another totally incapacitated for life as a result of the procedure. That's when the LeFever group stopped doing it."

Despite frequent and worrisome side effects, the procedure earned its originator, Antonio Moniz of Portugal, a 1949 Nobel Prize for Physiology or Medicine. And despite repeated tragic results, as Seymour witnessed, the procedure took years before it finally faded into obscurity.

"Later in my practice, I saw unnecessary sinus surgery, physicians putting burr holes in the skulls of headache patients, also called trephining or trepanning.

"Even the cardiologists were doing an interventional cardiac procedure on a condition where migraine patients have a patent ductus arteroisus, a heart defect in one-third of all patients where there is a shunt, or flow, between the two auricles of the heart. They'd pass a catheter into the heart, entering at the groin through the femoral vein, and then obliterate the hole between the auricles. Complicated migraines were treated this way.

"As rigid as the FDA rules are on the approval of medicines and despite their overwarnings that many times curtail the use of effective medicines, there is minimal or limited oversight on surgical procedures or devices used to help headache patients.

"I was soured at that point about neurosurgery and decided I would not want it as a career. Hippocrates said, 'I will prescribe regimens for the good of my patients according to ability and my judgment and *never do harm* to anyone.'"

Another disheartening episode intruded on Seymour's life at St. Mary's. He was assigned to examine the young girls who were slated to join the order of nuns.

"They were brainwashed, more or less. I don't think a girl of twelve knows how she wants to spend her life. It's not the devotion to religion that bothers me, just the idea of someone that young dedicating their life to anything at that age. Thank God things have changed nowadays."

On a lighter note, Seymour recalls comparing himself to one of Ivan Pavlov's canine test subjects, who were conditioned to salivate when they heard the bell rung, signaling that a tasty treat was imminent.

In Seymour's case, the bell was part of a system used to notify doctors when they were needed (replaced since by contemporary paging systems used in today's hospitals). A specific sequence of rings was assigned to each resident, and they often roused doctors from their between-patient naps in a room set aside especially for that purpose.

"My call was two short rings followed by a long one. I could be in a sound sleep, and they would be ringing the bell calls for any other doctor and it wouldn't wake me. But if the bell rang two shorts and a long, I would wake up immediately. I was like Pavlov's dog!"

So after a five- to six-month tenure at St. Mary's Hospital—as a full physician, by the way, not as an intern—Seymour planned his departure.

"I decided that I would come back to Chicago. I talked to the Mother Superior of the Order, and I told her I was unhappy, that I wanted to leave. She tried to dissuade me from leaving, but I told her I was pretty set on it.

"I discussed it with Elaine. She enjoyed her job, was very enthused with it, but she was willing to sacrifice what she was doing."

"Seymour hated surgery," Elaine confirms, "Just *hated* it! So, he knew he wasn't going to be a neurosurgeon, which is too bad because they're the princes of the field."

"Mother Superior sent me a wonderful note thanking me," Seymour adds, "and she included a hundred-dollar bill with it. That was so nice. That was a lot of money! She lauded me on my work ethic and my bedside manner with patients."

9. Back to Chicago and Home

C hicago in the year 1950 was a huge and prosperous city. Its population of 3.6 million marked the city's highest ever in history. (The 2010 census counted only 2.7 million residents.) A postwar building boom expanded into the suburbs and that, combined with growing automobile ownership, enabled development beyond the reach of mass transit lines.

Contributing to the city's population growth was the migration of African Americans from the South. Leaving behind Jim Crow laws and poor opportunity for advancement, black families headed north in search of jobs offered by WWII production during the conflict. Then, in the postwar years, plantation workers began their hopeful trips north in search of work when a cotton-picking machine replaced them in the fields.

Another draw was Chicago's South Side, which was claimed to be the "capital of black America." Earlier negotiations by the Congress for Industrial Organizations (CIO) in the 1930s had opened the doors to African Americans to work in the city's two largest industries, steel and meatpacking. For the first time, they were offered an opportunity not only to work, but to advance into management positions. To say that life was grand for black Americans in 1950s Chicago would be an exaggeration, however. They were still subject to discrimination in all its forms outside their South Side enclave.

Weather-wise, record summer temperatures scorched the city along with most of the Midwest in the 1950s, and five of Chicago's eleven hottest seasons occurred during the decade. According to records kept at Midway Airport, the '50s heat wave accounted for 276 days of temperatures above 90 degrees.

The only thing hotter than the sun was the music that thrived at such locations as the Blue Note jazz club, where bands—Benny Goodman, Duke Ellington, Count Basie—made the summers even hotter.

If the jazz was hot, the blues were cool, and the early 1950s framed the golden age of Chicago blues. Musicians upgraded from acoustic to electric guitars played over a solid drumbeat, as blues legends Howlin' Wolf and Muddy Waters played live in the clubs and recorded with a South Side company run by brothers Leonard and Phil Chess. Chess Records is remembered by many enthusiasts as it was described by musician/critic of the era, Cub Koda: "America's greatest blues label."

As rock 'n' roll began to replace jazz and blues among the younger generation's preferences, Chess Records would host such groups as the Rolling Stones in their recording studios. They would continue to evolve, and today the Chess library is owned by Universal Music Group and offered under the Geffen label.

The arts took a lively step into the future as well, described by art historian Peter Selz in an article titled "Surrealism and the Chicago Imagists of the 1950s: A Comparison and Contrast" as "eccentric and idiosyncratic." He continues: "Young Chicago artists shared with the Surrealists an interest in tribal, primitive, and exotic art, as well as the art of children and the insane."

Seymour's favorite baseball team, the Chicago White Sox, won sixty of their 154 games during the 1950 baseball season, placing sixth in the overall standings. (The New York Yankees won.) It was the Sox's fiftieth season as a team. Their home field was Comiskey Park, named after Charles Comiskey, who was first a player, then a manager, and finally the White Sox team owner. After his son, J. Louis Comiskey, passed away, his daughter-in-law, Grace, gained control of the team in 1950, passing it along to her daughter, Dorothy Comiskey Rigney, when Grace died in 1956.

Chicago mayor in 1950, Martin H. Kennelly was the son of a packinghouse worker, born in the city's Bridgeport neighborhood. Apparently he wasn't a strong leader, and the city council was said to have been running the city. One act in particular passed by the council backfired when they blocked the Chicago Housing Authority's bid to put housing projects in white neighborhoods as well as black. As a result, Chicago got the reputation of being the "most segregated city in the U.S."

In the '50s and '60s, the Chicago Housing Authority created eleven public housing projects which, although they apparently seemed a good idea at the time, isolated poor black single-parent families in so-called "superblocks" that were virtually impossible to patrol by the Chicago Police Department. Crime thrived, and the housing project failed.

After eight years in office, Mayor Kennelly's party abandoned him, perhaps due to its leadership by Richard Joseph Daley, who became Chairman of the Cook County Democratic Central Committee in 1953. Daley then became mayor in 1955 and would hold the office until his death in 1976.

On a national level, Harry S. Truman, a Democrat, was president, having succeeded to the presidency in 1945 when Franklin D. Roosevelt died while in office. Truman then won the election for his first full term in 1948.

Such was the Chicago, Illinois, USA, that Seymour and Elaine entered in 1950, their hopes high for a successful medical career and a home in which to raise a family.

Once again, the Flamms rose to the occasion, helping them move home from Cincinnati and get set up in Chicago. And once again, it wasn't easy, with housing to find and a practice to build.

First came the challenge of finding a place to live, but thanks again to Elaine's parents, that part wasn't so difficult.

Seymour recalls: "Her parents volunteered to have us stay with them. They had a nice three-bedroom apartment on the North Side near Lincoln Park. Most apartments—and even the one we have today— have two nice bedrooms and a maid's room. And when we came to live, I guess they moved Elaine's sister Barbara to the maid's room. She wasn't a happy camper over it, I'll tell you that!

"It served as temporary housing, I'd say at least for a year or a year and a half. Her mother and father couldn't have been nicer to us. Her father was a very intelligent man, and I really respected him.

He was a nice man. Her mother was a little more aggressive, and I didn't have the same feelings. But she was nice to us, and I always respected that. (She was a mixer. She mixed into people's business.)"

Seymour still had to take the Illinois State Board Exams to get his license to practice in the state, and he took two to three months to study for it.

"I took my state boards and passed them in the upper percentile," he recalls.

Decades later, he reminisces today, when he and Elaine purchased a winter home in Palm Springs, California, he decided to apply for his California license to practice. Part of the exam included an interview with two physicians who provided a series of tricky test questions.

By then he'd become well established as a headache specialist, and of course, his testers were aware of it. Seymour recalls what he refers to as a "curveball" question they tossed him.

"If you have a twenty-six-year-old woman with abdominal pain and vaginal bleeding, what would be your differential diagnosis?" they asked.

"Do you have any questions from the neck up?" he joked in response before giving them the correct answer: ectopic pregnancy. (It's a rare pregnancy complication where the embryo winds up in the wrong location, outside the uterine cavity, and typically in a fallopian tube.)

"They did not laugh," Seymour adds.

He passed the test, of course.

But back in 1950, none of this success had yet transpired, and he had to devise a way to convert his education with all its accompanying skills into a livelihood.

"If you wanted to go into general practice, you had to build the practice. And that's a slow process; maybe one patient would refer you his cousin and so on, but that's the way you built it. After I got the license, the next problem was to find an office location.

"I thought that the suburbs would be good because people were moving there. Skokie at that time was close to where we lived, Skokie and Evanston. Evanston was practically non-Jewish at all. And there was already a built-up community, so I didn't even attempt to go there.

Likewise with Skokie and Lincolnwood. I decided I would go out to a community that was growing very prosperously, Morton Grove.

"There was a pharmacy out there, and the pharmacist advertised a medical office for rent upstairs over his store. He wanted to lease it to a physician because he could prosper by it as well. If you've got a doctor upstairs or next door to you, people are going to fill their prescriptions with you."

It sounded like a promising opportunity, complete with a good working relationship with the pharmacist, and Seymour pursued it.

"I decided I would talk to him. I went out there, and we had a long talk. Then he said, 'You know, Dr. Diamond, I don't think this community is going to accept you. We're primarily a non-Jewish community. We don't have any Jews out here.'"

And so Seymour's search for an office space continued.

"I was looking at some other ads, and there was an ad for an office in Chicago near Bryn Mawr and Western. Elaine's father went out with me to look at it. It was on the second floor. There was a Jewish pharmacist down on the main floor, and there were apartments all around it.

"The fact that there was a Jewish pharmacy downstairs and a Jewish dentist nearby gave me a good feeling about it. I felt it would work out. One of the things that turned me away from it was its location. It was directly across from the main entrance to Rosehill Cemetery. It's one of the oldest cemeteries in Chicago, by the way."

In fact, the 350-acre Rosehill Cemetery was chartered in 1859, making it the oldest and largest nonsectarian graveyard in the city. Its present-day website claims more than a dozen Chicago mayors, four Illinois governors, and twelve Civil War generals as its permanent residents.

While Seymour didn't relish the idea of having 350 acres of deceased famous folk just across the street, he decided to open his practice there anyway.

"So the first thing I needed to do once I had my office was to find a hospital. If you're going into general medicine, you should affiliate with a hospital. I was about half a mile from Swedish Covenant. I went over there and talked to the administrator, and he told me that they have restrictions; they only have one Jew on the staff. Then I went to Ravenswood Hospital. It's no longer in existence today, but I was turned down there as well. Next I tried Columbus Hospital, but I was turned down there, too.

"Finally I went to Illinois Masonic, and they welcomed me. It was a big hospital and during my last year of medical school, I'd done some outpatient training there. So they knew me. And I established a case where I could hospitalize my patients. I received temporary privileges at first, then full privileges later."

At last, everything was in place for young doctor Diamond to run his general practice. Almost.

"I had an office, I had a hospital, but I had no patients! So, during those days, what did you do? I told the administrator, William Tenney, at Masonic that I was looking for patients, and he instructed his telephone operators that if anybody called the hospital without a doctor, that they would refer me some work. I also informed the dentist next door that I was looking for people and hoped maybe he could help me. But he was never any great help. And the same thing for the drugstore downstairs from my office, which should have been a fairly good source of help. Nothing."

Today most young doctors go directly into a medical group office rather start up their own office and find their own patients.

"Next, I contacted AT&T. It was different then; there was no 911 emergency service. Still, people would call for help, and they were very kind in referring me a lot of house calls. I didn't get paid on a lot of them, and a lot of them were in very bad neighborhoods, but it did me good in building up the practice. I'd meet new patients, and they referred other people to me. I was welcoming to anybody that would come at that time."

"There were no twenty-four-hour pharmacies in the whole city except for one. So I had the idea of going in and talking to the pharmacist there. And he started to refer me work.

"All these things helped stimulate the practice. You had to be creative in those days!"

Seymour's need for income while he was building his practice sometimes brought him to places where he didn't want to be ...

"I had heard that the Chicago Health Department was hiring part-time doctors. So I went down there and filled out an application, and they hired me. I was supposed to work three afternoons a week from 1:00 to 5:00 p.m. at one of the clinics. They primarily did immunizations at these clinics—whooping cough and diphtheria—all the diseases for which children get shots. I had plenty of time, and I could see plenty of patients privately on the other days. This job would give me some income while I was building my practice.

"At the clinics, I was supposed to examine each youngster, and then the nurse would give the injection. The first day, they sent me to an entirely African American community with somewhere over a hundred children. I started the exams, they started to give shots, and then the nurses who were giving the shots said to me, 'We'll be here until nine o'clock tonight. You can't examine them that carefully!' I was meticulous in my examinations despite the harassment from the nurses. I got out of there about seven or eight o'clock that night, and I went home to Elaine and said, 'You know, I don't think this is worth it.'

"It was like mass production. I didn't like it. So, I called in and told them I was going to quit the next day. I thanked them for giving me the job, but said that it wasn't for me.

"They asked me to come down to talk to them about my resignation. Dr. William Fishbein was second in command of the Chicago Board of Healthand an epidemiologist, and he wanted to talk to me personally. Political appointee Dr. Herman Bundesen officially oversaw the department as its president, but in practice, it was Dr. Fishbein.

"I went into his office, and he said, 'I see that you quit, but before I accepted your resignation, I looked at your application. I see that you were one of the editors of your medical school scientific publication.' And he said, 'I'd like you to keep your position. In fact, we're going to move you up a little bit here. We'd like you to stay with the Health Department, and we'll move up your status to a different classification.' I don't know what it was called, but it meant that I'd receive more money.

"He explained to me that Dr. Bundesen and he wrote a syndicated column under Dr. Bundesen's byline, and they needed somebody to write the articles for them. It was for a daily newspaper column called "Health—How to Keep It."

Seymour had enjoyed his editorial experiences in school, and he was confident in his medical knowledge. Now someone was offering him an opportunity to combine the two and get paid for it? He couldn't resist.

"My strengths in the library helped me. I would either go to the library or look at the journals. I'd look at their lead article and try to make it of interest to the general public. I would write the medical information, and then Elaine would edit it into wording a layman could read comfortably. Effie Alley from the old *Chicago Herald-Examiner* would stylize the column. Writing was a good source of income where I could devote myself to the practice without spending a lot of time away from it. I could write the column in the evening or over every weekend. I would do a week's worth and bring it in once a week."

Seymour worked with the Health Department ghostwriting columns for Dr. Bundesen when Chicago experienced its infamous horse meat scandal of 1952. Media coverage of the story was widespread. Both *Time* and *Life* magazines printed reports.

The headline read: "Chicago Rebels Against Filly de Mignon" in the February 11, 1952, issue of *Life* magazine and then continued with this colorful opening sentence: "The Hog Butcher of the World had a queasy stomach last week. The citizens of Chicago, who are wont to accept with blasé equanimity their gang wars, blizzards, the smell of the stockyards, their over-chlorinated drinking water, were shaken to their vitals by some news about their victuals."

Illinois racketeers were selling horse meat masquerading as beef, and it was being served in even the finest Chicago restaurants. The price of beef being four times that of the equine product, getting the meat past health inspectors involved bribery, and thus the departments, both local and state, were held accountable.

After confessing that he'd accepted $3,500 in bribes, Charles W. Wray, head of the Illinois Division of Foods and Dairies, was fired along with nine of his inspectors, and Chicago Board of Health Chief Food Inspector Gustav Hermann resigned under fire.

In early March of 1952, Illinois's Attorney General instructed his staff to indict Chicago Board of Health President Dr. Herman N. Bundesen for his department's part in the scandal, and although Dr. Bundesen stepped down from his position to deal with his court proceedings, Seymour continued his ghostwriting job.

Then, near the end of April, the criminal court threw out the indictment against Dr. Bundesen, and he returned to work in his former position. Seymour continued to write for the Health Department as he pursued his private practice, but eventually his Health Department position came to an end.

"Eight years into the job, there was an article in *JAMA*, the *Journal of the American Medical Association*, about antihistamines causing childhood deaths and that parents should be cautious not to give them overdoses.

"I wrote an article about it, and Dr. Bundesen called me in his office about a month later. He told me that a company that advertised heavily in all the Hearst newspapers where the "Health—How to Keep It" column was published had canceled all of their advertising because of my article. The company is not in existence today, by the way.

"From that point on he, or he and Dr. Fishbein together, began to carefully monitor every article that I wrote. No longer was it easy to bring them in on a Monday morning; I had to be about three months ahead of the publication date. I'd bring them in on Monday, and on Thursday they would send them back to me with a bunch of corrections. This never happened before. I would correct them, and by Monday, it would be corrected again!

"By that time, my practice was booming, and I said, 'You know, I'm going to leave.' I think they wanted me to leave, and it was fine with me at the time."

Refocused entirely on his own practice now, with Elaine working on the phones and as a receptionist, Seymour worked on as a general practitioner. And of course, he has a few stories from the experience.

"In 1954, I made a house call on a man about forty years old who had fainted. When I arrived, he was conscious but reported a history of four previous similar episodes. His heart rate was forty beats per minute (extremely low), and I hospitalized him. I phoned a professor of medicine at Chicago Medical School, Nathan Flaxman. Nate and I had sort of bonded in school, and the friendship extended into my family practice. Together, we made a diagnosis of Adams-Stokes syndrome, in which either heart block is slowing the heart or another cardiac condition is preventing adequate circulation to the brain. Jointly, we arrived at the conclusion that a medication that had not been previously used in these cases—methamphetamine—may benefit this particular patient. Fortunately, we were successful with this treatment and decided to publish an article on this case, 'The use of methamphetamine hydrochloride in Stokes-Adams disease.' It appeared in the *American Practitioner and Digest of Treatment* in 1955. Thus, a writing career was launched!

"As an aside to this story, in October of 2009, I was lecturing in Chicago at the Diamond Headache Clinic Research & Education[al] Foundation's seventh annual research summit. About ten minutes into my lecture, I turned pale and fainted—an episode of Stokes-Adams. After careful monitoring for about one week, the diagnosis was heart block, and a pacemaker was inserted into my chest to regulate my heartbeat. The procedure proved successful as I have had no further episodes," Seymour added.

"When I was making calls from Illinois Masonic Hospital, William Tenney, who was the administrator for the hospital, caught me one day as I was coming in to see one of my patients. He said, 'A man called in and told me that his wife was very, very sick. I know you're coming here to see a couple patients and you want to get to your office, but we like to take care of the people in the neighborhood. Would you do me a favor and go over there and see her?'

"So I drove over to a little bungalow about eight blocks from Illinois Masonic. I found the man, who said, 'Oh, doctor, I'm glad you're here. Come up and see my wife. She is so, so sick.'

"So I went into the bungalow, and he took me into his bedroom. And there was an empty bed!

"I didn't know what to do. I asked him how long she'd been sick and he says, 'She's been in bed for six, seven, eight months, and she hasn't been able to move.'

"I said, 'Is she in the washroom?'

"And he says 'No. She's right there in bed. Can't you see her?'

"Well, I still wasn't sure what to do, but I took out my mercury thermometer, shook it, and pretended to take her temperature. I did likewise with her blood pressure. Next, I took out my stethoscope and pretended to listen, and then I said, 'I think this will improve as time goes on.'

"And he says, 'Well, can I pay you?'

"And I said, 'No, the hospital asked me to come, so let's just call it even.'

"I drove away and subsequently informed the hospital about it, that apparently he was having delusions and needed some psychiatric care."

Another case early in his career confirmed Seymour's belief in God. He was at his home in Evanston, a colonial-style house in a quiet neighborhood, on a Sunday morning doing weekend chores and spending time with his family.

"About 1:00 p.m., I got a call from a patient of mine. They were a young couple in their late twenties. His wife called to tell me her husband was experiencing tremendous chest pains and having difficulty breathing.

"I sent him into the hospital and had the emergency room physician examine him. They ran an EKG, which was normal. Blood tests to detect coronary artery disease were not available at that time. However, my instincts told me that we should probably admit him and observe him overnight.

"I was home working on our lawn, taking out the crabgrass, setting up my sprinklers, and other chores, as I would typically do on a Sunday. I had a casual dinner with my family and then drove to the hospital to see him.

"I went to his room, and I had them do another EKG while I was there. I waited and looked at it. It was perfectly normal. His in-laws and his wife were there, and I reassured them that everything was okay and that they should go home, which they did.

"I went up to the desk to write a progress note on the patient's chart. I want to say that Sunday night is the worst night to be sick in a hospital because it's really—then, anyway—the most undermanned night. So I wrote the progress note, and normally, I would have just written the note and left because I had no reason to go back.

"But I didn't leave. Instead, I walked back to his room. I had no medical or other logical reason to do that. I just had a feeling that I should. And as I walked into the room, he experienced a complete cardiac arrest!

"I jumped up on the bed and began giving him CPR and yelling for help. He had a massive heart attack, and if I hadn't been right there, I don't know if he would have survived. As it turned out, he came through the whole thing in perfect health.

"Something guided me that night. To me, the circumstances of how and what I did that day impressed on me that some higher force or knowledge was guiding me to return to that man's room, exactly when and where I was needed to save his life."

While Seymour was affiliated with Illinois Masonic Hospital, he gained the respect and friendship of eminent pathologist Dr. Lester King. Dr. King later went on to become the book editor for the American Medical Association, and when it came time to review books dealing with headache or pain in general, he'd send them along to Seymour. "I was honored to do all the book reviews on headache and pain from 1974 through 1976," Seymour recalls.

It was also during his time with Illinois Masonic Hospital that Seymour joined theAncient Egyptian Arabic Order Nobles of the Mystic Shrine, also known as the Shriners. Apparently it was the thing to do in that environment, and he felt it necessary to forward his career while working there.

The North Park Hotel in Chicago featured expansive suites where out-of-town actors, singers, and other performers liked to stay when they were in town, and occasionally they needed medical care.

"I met the telephone operator for the hotel, and she asked me if I would like to be the doctor for the hotel. She introduced me to the hotel manager and he approved. They had several more hotels, so I would take calls for about three or four of the smaller hotels. I built up a fairly good practice with these patients, although they were transient and unlikely to return after they'd left the city.

"But some of the actors were in shows that lasted for six months or a year, and they would become longer-term patients. For example, the show *South Pacific* was in Chicago at that time. Over a four- or five-month period, I saw many of the cast repeatedly.

"George Gaynes, a prominent singer in a musical that was playing in Chicago, was one of my patients. One day he walked in without an appointment, and I was busy. I told him it would be at least a half hour. I was always very punctual about appointments.

"So, he said, 'I'm going to walk across the street and look around.' Remember, I was across the street from the Rose Hill Cemetery.

"I had never been in the cemetery. When he came back and after I had taken care of him, he's the one who told me about all the people who helped form Chicago who were laid to rest there. He was a very interesting man."

George Gaynes was born George Jongejans in Finland, although he spent most of his life in the United States. Under his original family name, he became a successful opera singer on the stages of Italy and France before World War II and in the U.S. afterward. To most of us, he's better known as the curmudgeonly Henry Warnimont in the TV series *Punky Brewster* or Commandant Lassard in the first of seven *Police Academy* movies.

Gaynes's drop-in appointment reminds Seymour to tell us about his beliefs on keeping appointments: "It has always been my policy to keep appointments at the appointed time. It wasn't always possible, but I thought it was an affront to a patient to keep them waiting too long.

"I've always tried to teach this to various doctors that have worked under me or been associated with me. And they never listen. I worked for everything I had, and I think a lot of these kids coming up don't appreciate what they have or how they got it."

In addition to appointment punctuality or lack thereof, Seymour wants to talk about fee splitting.

"In the years when I first got into medicine, there was an accepted practice of fee splitting. In other words, the general practitioner would get maybe $10 for the call, but when he hospitalized a patient who had an appendectomy, the surgeon would get a big fee. We're talking about $300 to $400, but that was a lot of money in those days. The surgeon would give a rebate back to the referring physician. The ethics of the practice were questioned, and such arrangements became outlawed maybe twenty years after I was in practice," Seymour recalls.

"It's considered unethical in the profession today. The American College of Surgeons eliminated it in the late 1960s."

In the late 1950s, Seymour became fascinated with the new and upcoming field of nuclear medicine.

"There were college courses I could take, but my practice was so busy I couldn't do that. But one of the founders of the Cook County Hospital Nuclear Medicine department was a doctor who had a severe muscular or neurological tremor. He was a pioneer, and he agreed (I was very persistent then) to give a series of lectures. He devised a course so people could learn about nuclear medicine, and I spent my Wednesdays going to his classes for about six months.

"Subsequent to that, a small society of nuclear medicine was formed, and I was accepted as a member because I had actually had some training, both academically and in practice. I saw a future in it, and now, it's a separate specialty in medicine.

"But I had an interest in it, and I thought it had a place in my practice. In coordination with that, the pharmaceutical industry was doing studies where they tagged a drug with an isotope. You can trace it and measure the half-life.

"I bought some equipment, a lot of it funded by the research I was doing. I think it was carbon-14, which is the tagged molecule that we used. I did a number of tests during that time for various pharmaceutical houses, and it was very interesting work.

"I used it therapeutically in my family practice. One of the specific early uses was for hyperthyroidism. It was at that time, anyway, more prominent and frequent than it is now. Iodine was the drug typically used, but sometimes the iodine fails and it's cumbersome. Giving a tagged isotope will usually burn it out. It's a way of convenient treatment, and I started to use it in practice. I received referrals because people knew I was able to do it, but that stopped as my headache work started to materialize.

"Here are a couple of anecdotes: You had to have a locked, lead-shielded safe for storage of the radioactive materials. You could store it for a few days, but after a week, it would no longer be potent. You needed fresh material. It'd be flown in, protectively sealed in lead-lined containers, and it has a certain half-life. So you couldn't just store it until you needed it. You could store it for a few days and measure the half-life, but that was it.

"I had a federal license to do this, although I don't know if you need it today. Its use was primarily for thyroid disease at that time, research, and they used radioactive rods to treat certain cancers, primarily cancer of the cervix or uterus. The rods were the potent things and had a long half-life.

"We were subject to an inspection at will, and usually they came around every three months. What they did was test the area with a Geiger counter to make sure there wasn't any exposure. They would also do an extensive inventory of your radioactive material.

"One of the inspectors was inspecting our facility at about 11:00 a.m., so I took him to lunch. Usually federal employees don't do this, but he had a sandwich, and we were talking. And he said he had just done an inspection in a hospital in Missouri, a large city in Missouri, so I presume it was St. Louis, but he didn't say so specifically.

"And when he did an inventory of their safe, some of the radioactive rods were missing!

"They did an investigation. It was within a hospital, and they had a large radiology department, so they questioned all the technicians. They checked the records of where it was used, and then they decided to do a Geiger counter search.

"They tested the office, the treatment areas, and everywhere else, and finally they went to the radiologist's office. And the Geiger counter started to click like mad! It clicked loudly, and then started to intensify when they came to the radiologist's chair. And there it was so loud they knew they had found something.

"Buried in the fabric of his chair were three rods! Apparently he was having an affair with one of the technicians, but then broke it off. And this was her revenge!"

By now, Seymour's practice was going well, and he decided to make up for an earlier miscue.

"I never gave Elaine a diamond ring because I couldn't afford it when we became engaged," Seymour begins. "It was very important to me. I had a good friend who was in the diamond business, Chuck Milner, but I didn't buy it from him. He was a friend and a wholesaler, and I didn't want to depreciate the gift to her by getting it cheaply.

"There was a very famous jeweler on Michigan Avenue in the Drake Hotel. So, I went in there and told the salesman I wanted as clear a stone as he could give me. I told him how many carats I wanted, and I told him I wanted an exceptionally white color to it. With his help, I picked out a ring for Elaine and surprised her with it.

"Then, Elaine's mother, Bessie, after she got the ring, kept saying to Elaine that she should get it appraised. I told her, 'Look, I insured it, I sent the sales slip in with it, and I think it takes away from the gift to appraise it.' I argued. I didn't want to do it.

"But after much insistence by her mother, we took it in to the diamond appraisers in a special jewelry building, and we had it appraised. And the appraiser said it had a lot of flaws, it had poor color ... nothing like I expected.

"So then I asked my friend Chuck Milner if he would look at it. He concurred in the appraiser's diagnosis. So, I called the salesman and told him I would like to return the ring because of the appraisal, but he said, 'We don't take things back.'

"I didn't know what to do. The only general lawyer I knew was Harold Levine, my brother-in-law, and he said, 'You don't want a lawsuit,' which was good advice. I don't like lawsuits anyway. Then he said, 'Go in there, and try to return it. And if they don't want to take it back, get in an argument and raise your voice!'

"And sure enough, they took it back and gave me a check refund. It wasn't bad. I raised my voice a little bit. Harold said to be sure to go there at a busy time, and they had a lot of customers in there when I complained.

"Then I went to my friend Chuck Milner. He sold me a beautiful ring, and we've been very happy with it. I just didn't go to him first because I thought it would take away the significance of the gift. Going wholesale was not what I wanted to do. I didn't care if I paid a little more for it."

Much later in life, Seymour decided to buy a piece of fine jewelry for himself, a watch, and his friend-in-the-business Chuck Milner helped him then, too.

"On my sixtieth birthday, Elaine and I talked, and I decided that I wanted a special watch for myself. And I sort of predetermined what I wanted to buy. But Elaine thought we should look at a watch store to see what available. We happened to be in New York when we were discussing it. I was giving a talk there, and there's a fine watch store known as Tourneau.

"I decided I wanted the 18K gold Rolex. But before I bought it, I went to my friend Chuck Milner and asked his advice about the Rolex. He told me it's a wonderful watch; however, you can't get any kind of a deal on it. The dealer will lose the Rolex franchise if they undercut the price, so it's full retail or nothing.

"But Chuck said if he were buying it for himself, since he's in the jewelry business, he has reciprocal agreements that provide a considerable discount. We're very close friends with Chuck and his wife, and so he bought the watch for me.

"On my way home one day, he called me and said, 'I have your watch, Seymour.' He lived in Lincolnwood, and I was living in the Skokie-Evanston area, so I said, 'I'll be coming home about five o'clock. What time will you be home?' He told me a little later than that, so I said, 'I'll work a little bit on some paperwork at the office, and I'll come by and pick it up.'

"I picked up the watch and put it on, and I said, 'Chuck, this is exactly what I wanted. In fact, it fits me better than the watch I tried on at Torneau." I thanked him and went home.

"No sooner did I get home than he called me and said, 'Seymour, I'm going to come by and pick up the watch.'

"I was shocked and said, 'Why, Chuck?'

"'Don't ask me any questions,' he replied, and he picked up the watch. A day later, he called me to say, 'I have your watch for you.' So, I went and picked it up again, just like I did before, and he gave me an envelope with two of the watchband links in it. It's all solid gold, you know.

"He said, 'The watch you got was short two links.' At that time, they were worth $250 each. I would never have realized it, and nobody else buying a Rolex would have realized it. Each of those links is worth about $1,500 today!"

10. The Kids

Seymour and Elaine raised three daughters, and each became another Diamond family success story in her own right.

Judi was born in 1951 as Seymour and Elaine were still settling in Chicago and building his medical practice. Seymour was twenty-six years old at the time, and Elaine was twenty-four. Until their first daughter was born, Elaine had spent her time helping Seymour get his practice off the ground by managing his office. After her first child was born, she became a stay-at-home mom.

Judi became an architect. She started college at the University of Michigan, where she met future husband Nathan Falk, who was studying to become a lawyer. They became a couple, and when Nate went to law school in Chicago, Judi also transferred to a school in the Windy City. The artist in the Diamond family, she first earned her undergraduate degree majoring in psychology with a minor in fine arts from Northwestern University. The degree was presented "with distinction" since she would have graduated Phi Beta Kappa, but that option wasn't available to her because she'd transferred from Michigan. She went to the Art Institute of Chicago and became a graphic designer and printmaker, working for years doing lithography and etchings.

Eventually, Judi and Nate made the decision to have children, and with that decision came a change in her career path. The chemicals used in Judi's work were toxic, unsafe around the kids, and not good for expectant mothers. She decided architecture would be a good alternative and earned her master's degree at the University of Illinois. Nate, who had been working as a public defender, started his own trial law firm so that he could spend more time with his family, helping care for the kids as Judi studied.

She founded Diamond-Falk Architects, Inc., in 1996 to provide architectural design, planning, consultation, and construction management as well as interior and furniture design. Awards include an award for restoration given jointly by the Evanston Preservation Commission and the Preservation League of Evanston for her own single family home, where she and husband Nathan Diamond-Falk raised their family.

Judi has helped Seymour design his various office spaces and his living quarters in Chicago and in Palm Springs. She manages a variety of residential and commercial projects with the support of her team.

Daughter number two, Merle, was born in 1954.

Merle became a doctor, following in her dad's footsteps. She attended the University of Michigan for her premedical education, graduating with high honors, and then attended Northwestern University in Evanston, Illinois, for medical school.

"I'd been accepted at a number of medical schools," Merle recalls today, "but Dad wanted me to go to the one he felt would provide me with best education, which was Northwestern. He didn't mind about the cost. He was very generous that way. He wanted me to have the best."

She recalls her dad's support when interviewing at the various schools: "My dad came with me. That was a really wonderful experience!"

Merle completed her residencies in emergency medicine/internal medicine at McGaw Medical Center of Northwestern University. Since then, she earned subspecialty certification for Headache Medicine from the United Council for Neurologic Subspecialties. She is a former member of the American College of Emergency Physicians and currently is a diplomat of the American Board of Internal Medicine.

Although she liked the challenge and variety that emergency medicine provided, after being physically assaulted ("kicked across the room") by a patient while pregnant with her son Michael, she left the ER behind and moved fulltime into headache medicine in

1989 at her dad's Diamond Headache Clinic. She works there today as president and managing director.

Third daughter, Amy, was born in 1958.

Amy became a journalist. She studied at the University of Michigan, receiving her B.A. in journalism from the College of Literature, Science, and the Arts. She went to work in Wisconsin at Milwaukee's the Journal Company as a staff reporter at the *Milwaukee Sentinel* from 1980 to 1984 before returning to Chicago to attend Northwestern University's Medill School of Journalism. At Northwestern, she earned her master of science degree in journalism in 1985.

After leaving Northwestern with her master's degree, she worked for Consumers Digest, Inc., in Chicago as Senior Editor (promoted from Associate Editor) for *Money Maker* magazine.

Amy moved to Los Angeles in 1988 and found employment at Petersen Publishing Company, first as a copy editor, then as the editorial production manager for *Sport Truck* and *Circle Track* magazines.

She left Petersen for a brief stint at Toyota Motor Sales, U.S.A., Inc., in Torrance as corporate publications editor in 1989–1990 and at Pacific Magazine Group in Malibu, California, as managing editor of *Presentation Products* magazine before returning to Petersen Publishing Company as managing editor of *4-Wheel & Off-Road* and *Rod & Custom* magazines.

From that point on, she grew within the company, serving as group operations manager for the Truck Division from 1991–1994, group operations manager for the TEEN Magazine Group from 1994–1996 when Robert E. Petersen sold his 50-year-old, privately-owned publishing company to an investment group.

The publishing company was sold four times altogether: next to Emap USA, a British-owned magazine publisher; then to Primedia, Inc.; and finally to the current owner, Source Interlink Media, LLC.; and each time Amy earned her niche in the new management team. Her current position with Source Interlink Media is vice president of editorial operations.

Along the way, she also helped the Diamond Research & Educational Foundation as an editorial consultant for its publication *Headache Quarterly*, and coauthored several books with her dad, including *Headache and Your Child*, *Headache and Diet*, and *Hope for Your Headache Problem*.

So, what was it like growing up as Seymour and Elaine's children?

"Our family life was pretty normal," Judi begins. "I was first, and so probably my picture was different. I felt they were really pretty strict with me, so I kind of made it easier for my sisters by testing the waters, was my feeling on it."

The youngest, Amy, agrees: "By the time they got to me, I think they had seen everything, and I didn't have a lot of restrictions. Fortunately, I imposed my own limits. I think we're all kind of wild. Maybe Judi wasn't. She was gone by the time I was growing up, so they probably were a bit stricter with her. But it was a different era, too, so. Not that she's that much older, but I think I definitely got to do a lot more than either of them. Just because they had all done it already and by the time they got to me, it was like, 'Well, I'm sure she'll turn out fine.'"

"Right," Judi nods. "I mean, they babied her a lot. You know, and she was everybody's little baby. So, we all kind of spoiled her."

"I remember my freshman year in high school," Merle interjects. "I think for my first semester I got straight Bs, and Judi was applying for college at the time. I think they asked her to have a talk with me, that I wouldn't get into any schools with that kind of a performance. The message was sent; that wasn't acceptable.

"I was very competitive with Judi, and I figured anything she could do, I could do. So I just figured out a way to get good grades."

"I think Amy and I were alike more than Merle," Judi continues, "because there was such an age difference, and in looking at three girls … there's competition. I think our family had a lot of competition. I think everybody (and again, this is just my opinion), but you know, there was one man and four women. I think everybody competed for my father's attention, and he wasn't there very much.

"They tried to have dinner together as a family a lot, and that was important, but otherwise, he was really busy with work. And then at night they'd go play bridge a lot. So, we'd have a sitter. My recollection is that dinner tables and family things were fairly loud. We were competing for attention."

At the mention of the sitter, Amy adds, "Mrs. Hanson! Oh, Mrs. Hanson was the best! She was a patient of my dad's when he was in general practice, and I guess he hired her to babysit the kids, mostly me.

"I just loved Mrs. Hanson. She taught me how to bake. She was a fabulous baker, just fabulous. We used to make beef Stroganoff and play card games like UNO … and Candyland, when I was younger. We just had a great time! She had the best personality; a happy, happy woman.

"She was truly more—I hate to say this, but—more a grandmother to me than either of my grandparents. I just loved Mrs. Hanson! She would always invite me over at Christmas time to help her and her husband, Carl, decorate their tree. It was so much fun!

"And then her husband passed away, but she lived quite long. I remember she was born in 1900, and that was always such a big thing to me. I think she lived until she was ninety-something. I got to meet her grandkids and members of her family

"I definitely liked when Mrs. Hanson sat for me more than my dad's nurses. I didn't like when they stayed with us when my parents would go on trips. There were a couple of evil ones. I don't even remember who they were, but they weren't very nice. I don't have great memories of that, but I also wasn't happy when my parents went away either. I hated separation from them, even if I had to go to religious school, and I used to cry like a baby when my mom would drop me off places. I didn't think they'd come back."

Sometimes, as Judi and Merle entered high school, they'd babysit for their little sister. "I was the baby," Amy reminds us. "I always had to do whatever my sisters said. You know, I covered for them a lot when they were babysitting me and had people over at the house. They'd take me out, get me ice cream. They bribed me. But you know, I think that's typical big sister, little sister stuff."

Amy is a lifelong dog lover, currently caring for Scout, a five-year-old female yellow Labrador retriever, and Groovy, a male, four-and-a-half-year-old brindle-colored Bouvier des Flandres, and she remembers her childhood pets with love.

"We had two dogs, poodles named Mocha and Collette. Mocha was Merle's dog, and he was mean. Collette was Judi's and my dog, and she was sweet. Mocha would bite people. When my mom would come in to say goodnight to us (Merle and I shared a room), Mocha would growl and try to bite. But he always did that. He was just kind of a mean dog.

"We got them from one of my dad's patients, Mary Bak, who bred poodles. I remember we'd go to her house. It was in the city, and her house would just be filled with poodles! It was fun to go there!

"One day, one of my dad's patients gave him a Great Dane as a present. We couldn't keep him—he was huge—so he gave the Great Dane to Mary Bak. So she had all these poodles and a Great Dane, who they named Seymour, of course."

Merle adds, "I loved animals. I got a mynah bird. I don't know how I talked them into it, but I did. And then I got a snake. My mother hated all of those things. And then I had a sore throat or something, and my father used to come home and give us shots. He was a bad shot giver, and I think he must have hit a blood vessel or something. I had some bleeding, not serious, and I negotiated them into getting the dog. So when I came home from summer camp, we went and picked up Mocha."

Judi picks up the conversation again: "I got married at nineteen, and I think that the thing I really adored about Nate Falk was how calm and laid-back he was. It was very different from my family. At the time I'm not sure I realized it, but there was a lot of pressure, a lot of pressure to succeed as well. As you can see, we all did these driven professions.

"It took a while for me to find the thing that I liked. Medicine just didn't seem to cut it for me. I wasn't that interested. But I did try. At first, when I applied to the University of Michigan, it was in nursing. But it didn't interest me in the least.

"I transferred out of nursing really quickly, but I stayed at Michigan for two years. I had met Nate right at the beginning, and then I transferred to Northwestern University in Evanston. Nate graduated, but he didn't get into law school at Michigan, so he went here in Chicago at DePaul University.

"I always liked art as I was growing up. But it's a hard thing to just say, that's what you're going to do. In junior high, I designed the yearbook and I was given things to do. However, I don't know … sometime in high school I seemed to have a teacher that didn't like what I did. When you're young, you're very influenced by those things."

Given Elaine and Seymour's extensive art collection today, we wondered how they may have influenced Judi's interest.

"They really did collect," she responds, "but it was much more realistic in those days. I think the appreciation for the arts was there, and they never discouraged me from going into the arts. It's just that in my own mind, I felt that going into medicine was what they wanted. Or what my father wanted. But I'm not sure … it could have just been my perception of it. And then when Merle decided to do that, it was kind of a relief.

"I think nowadays as parents, we get more involved in what our kids do and what they're good at and helping them in their direction. At least I feel like we did a little more of that with our kids. We were really involved, and I guess it was a reaction, too. You know, it was really important to me that Nate wanted to be very involved in our kids' lives before we had kids. And I think it was a reaction to the fact that my father really wasn't. Although it was a different age, so you can't really criticize that. But before we decided to have children—we were married for seven or eight years before our son, Brian, was born—we had talked and we weren't sure we wanted to have children even. But whatever, we would do this together. I guess it's kind of a reaction—you end up running your life based on what you saw, either as for it or against it."

Judi's architecture skills were appreciated by her dad, and she would ultimately design a number of his offices, create his hospital in-patient units, and enhance his and Elaine's living quarters.

She found him easy to work with on all projects, particularly the home remodeling. She was the expert in such things, and Seymour was not. So, he relied on her good judgment and approved the work often without question or additional input.

Working with the hospital jobs was another story, not because of any issues Seymour would have, but with the hospitals' facility managers. In fact, she was quite helpful when dealing with them, acting as Seymour's advocate when his wishes and the facility managers' wishes conflicted.

"It was always a struggle," she recalls, "because I was dealing with hospital facility managers. Part of the reason I think he wanted me to do it was because I was much more of a residential architect, and he wanted his floors to look more residential. He needed an advocate because a lot of them had double rooms first, and we tried to get all singles. In dealing with facility managers, they don't really understand. They're more 'money people.' They'd like their rooms to be multipurpose.

"So it was always a struggle to try to get what the Headache Clinic wanted, or what my clients wanted. I was really working for the hospital; they paid the bills. As with anything, you work with your clients as to what they'd like. But in this case, I was being paid by the hospital but trying to design what the Diamond Headache Clinic wanted for their in-patient care facility. So, yes, it was sometimes a struggle."

Amy has also helped her dad in his medical work, using her journalism skills to coauthor several books with him. When first asked how she liked working with Seymour, she (thinking of her brief stint answering phones at the clinic) replied, "Oh, horrible. Well, the books were easier because that's my area of expertise. He could dictate or send me material and I'd just edit, rewrite, whatever it took, and that was fine.

"When I worked in the office, it was not fun. He's very demanding, and he can sort of be gruff sometimes without intending to be when he wants something. And you know, I just didn't think it was a good thing to work there. It did give me money, and it gave me a working experience. But, let's just say I liked working and dealing with people, but not really my boss. But I was fortunate because it did give me some working experience and organizational skills. I knew I would never go into medicine, so it definitely didn't pique my interest there."

Here Judi was asked to list her dad's good and bad traits.

"He's a very warm and giving person, friendly and open, and loyal, very loyal. Like a puppy dog. Unless you really wrong him. I think that those are really good traits. He'd do anything for you."

And his bad traits?

"Well, I think he has a really bad temper. And he's a little *controlling*. I'm saying it nicely, but there's probably a bit of that in all of us. I imagine for Merle it probably was a lot tougher because she worked in the same field. For Amy and me, we're in different fields, so it was easier."

On the positive side, Merle says, "I think he's a great clinician. He loves patients. He's an advocate for his patients. He has a passion for whatever he's interested in, a tremendous passion, and he's incredibly creative. He's a fount of information; he has encyclopedic knowledge. He'll see something and he'll be able to tell you, 'Oh, there's an article on that; it was written thirty years ago.' He has a vision of health care that we should strive for, and I think that's an amazing thing. He's taught me a tremendous amount. As a business partner, he's a little more problematic."

In response to the same questions, Amy first lists Seymour's good traits: "Oh, he's just the friendliest person on earth. He'll talk to anybody. He's dedicated. He's caring. He's inquisitive. He's generous to a fault. And he's smart, a very astute businessman. He reads a lot. I mean he really just absorbs things and understands them. He's just a sweetheart."

As for his "bad" traits, Amy responds, "Impatience. Kind of demanding. If I came home with an A-minus, he'd ask, 'Why didn't you get an A?' Or a B-plus, and he'd say, 'Why didn't you get an A-minus?' He was very, very focused on us doing well. That's about it for negatives.

"I just want to say I think all my good traits—especially when it comes to dealing with people—come from him. All the nice Midwestern things: friendliness, inquisitiveness, and caring about people … developed from him. I think that's the best thing he could ever have given me, as opposed to being book smart or anything. Just being a really good human being."

Nate and Judi provided Seymour and Elaine with their first grandchild, Brian Diamond-Falk. Elsewhere in this book, you'll read how Seymour had wanted the child named in a Jewish traditional ceremony and how he had arranged it.

Judi responds, "Yes, he did hire a rabbi. That's an example of his controlling things. You know, we have some of our own certain ideas. We did go along it, but we insisted there be no mention of a god. So, we were a little flexible at times. Those things weren't important to us particularly."

Judi and Nate Diamond-Falk welcomed daughter Emily to their family three years after Brian's arrival.

"You know, before she was born, I was praying that Emily would be a girl," Judi confides, "so there'd be no competition. I really wanted one of each and that was it! I didn't want three of anything."

"Katie, my daughter-in-law, grew up with three girls, and they're very close. No problems. They're best friends. But it just depends, and the only thing I can think of is a competition sort of thing. It was pretty intense at times."

As Seymour and Elaine's family grew larger, their house in the Budlong Woods area of Chicago grew smaller, and the Diamonds began looking for a new home. Like most of us, they wanted good schools for their children, a good value in their investment, and a comfortable neighborhood.

"We moved when Judi was about six years old because we wanted our kids to go to a good school system," Seymour begins. "Skokie-Evanston is the area where we wanted to move, so we looked at several houses in northwest Evanston. But we were discouraged from even making an offer on any of them because of our religion. Still, we wanted our children to attend the Evanston school system because of its excellent reputation.

"After we looked in Evanston, we looked at a lot of older houses. They were built by a contractor known as Hemphill. They were lovely houses, and he was the noted builder in that area. But we were discouraged from buying there, so then we went into Skokie. There's a special area there called Devonshire, and we bought a beautiful corner lot!

"We decided we'd build on it, but meanwhile, we saw an older Hemphill house for sale in the Skokie-Evanston area. It was a very mixed area ethnically with prominent Catholic, Protestant, and some Jewish people. It was a nice area.

"We liked the location, and there was a beautiful lot for sale there. We called the people that had it, and it was the Hemphill people—they owned the lots there, and the condition to buy it is that they would build the house for you.

"So we bought the lot. It was quite reasonable in comparison to the other one we bought. So I'm sitting on two lots and our old house in the Budlong Woods section of Chicago.

"We went to their architect, a very nice man, and he drew up plans for us. We had multiple meetings with him, and in the meanwhile, whenever we saw a house for sale on a Sunday, we would go out and look at it to get ideas.

"That was when we saw a house that we actually bought on Springfield Avenue. It was everything that we wanted him to build, and meanwhile, his bids were coming up at that time almost $30,000 above that house that was for sale. So, I made an offer of what I could afford on that house. We bought it, and it was a wonderful house.

"But now I'm sitting on two lots, the house in Chicago, and a house I just bought!

"I went to Devonshire, I had a sign made, drove it in, and in two days, I sold that lot. It was so fast, and I got double my price on it.

"Then, it was Mother's Day, and I got a call from the people in Chicago who were handling the sale of our old home. They had an offer. It was a lot less than I thought we should get, but I said, 'Fine. We're out.' I was strapped. I owned a lot of stuff all of the sudden. But I was willing to take the gamble.

"Then I called Hemphill, apologized to them, and said, 'Send me the architect's bills. I would like to sell the lot back to you.'

"So, I'm sitting with this beautiful lot, and I never got an architect's bill. I called several times and wrote to them that I would like to return it at the same price I paid for it. That was nice for them because it was worth a lot more by now. Still, no answer.

"Finally, I asked my lawyer brother-in-law Hank Levine what to do. He told me to send them a ninety-day notice. Tell them that they can redeem it, and if not, you're going to sell it.

"They never redeemed it, so then I sold it for more than what I paid for it. I just don't understand why they never redeemed it. I guess it was insignificant to them. But I never knew why for sure."

And so the Diamonds settled into their new home on Springfield Avenue in Skokie-Evanston. Seymour, never one to be idle, became involved in local politics when he was voted in as president of the Northeast Skokie Property Owners' Association, a position that became even more political than one might expect.

"Evanston, during that period, had a school board and superintendent that thought they should integrate the school. There were smaller sections within Skokie-Evanston. One was called Williamsburg Village, and the other was New England Village, like little villages with about forty or so homes in them.

"In this redistricting, five young white children would be going to an otherwise completely black school. Their parents came to me, as president, to go to a public meeting and speak up for them. So I went to the public meeting on it, and there were a lot of Jewish liberals around, and I spoke up for the five families. It was my job. I was president of the organization.

"I won my point, but I never got so much venom from the white liberals. They were very critical and even called me names. It just enhanced my conservative thoughts, though.

"One other story. The village of Skokie never did fireworks, so our organization decided that we would get permission and do fireworks at a little park in our area. We also had somebody come with horses and buggies to give rides to the children. I arranged it all.

"And it was funny—I was president at the time we did it—and I got a lot of nice calls and notes on it. But that evening when I got home, one of the neighbors who lived near the park called me and asked me who's going to clean up the horse manure! I guess he thought I was going to go out there with a shovel or something. I called city hall and got it handled."

From 1965 through 1968, Seymour served as president of the Skokie Board of Health at the request of friends who felt his influence would be beneficial.

"I told them I didn't want to be political in any way," he explains, "and if they were going to be political with me, I would resign. I don't believe that health should have anything to do with politics.

"The Skokie Health Department didn't have full recognition as a public health department because they didn't have a full-time physician who was knowledgeable in public health. And one of the things I wanted to achieve as its president was for it to become recognized. So, I recruited a physician from the Philippines who had the credentials to be the head of the department.

"There were about eight employees besides the physician. After he was there about two months, I got a call at my clinic from his assistant that everybody had resigned!

"So I drove back to Skokie to see if I could find out what was happening. And apparently, his method in handling employees was not the greatest. He had called a meeting of his employees and said, 'You,' (he called some of their names) and said, 'You are the good guys. You sit over here.' And then he called the names of the rest of the employees and he said, 'You sit on this side. You're the bad employees.'

"So I spent about an hour talking to them all and then talking to him, that he couldn't do things like that. It wasn't a proper method of handling employee relations. I said if there was ever any criticism, it would be better to let me know. I'd normally go to an evening meeting, and if they had a problem during the day, they would call me.

"Then after a few years, they started to nominate physicians who were politically connected to be on the board, which was really not going to help the public. So, I wrote a resignation letter and left the job for someone else."

Seymour left the presidential position displeased with the political maneuvers, but he had accomplished his goal of providing the city of Skokie with a full-time health department.

In June 1967, Seymour presented an exhibit at an American Medical Association Annual Convention titled, "The Family Physician Treats the Psychiatric Patient." He and colleague Dr. Irvin Belgrade won a gold medal for the effort, which was presented at the meeting by Dr. Verne L. Schlaser of Des Moines, along with a check for $100.

Seymour says that he postponed a family trip to Europe by a day so he could accept the award, adding that the airline had no problem working with him to make the change, a far cry from today's travel standards.

When Seymour and Elaine traveled abroad for medical meetings, they'd bring the girls along, too. Amy shares her memories of them.

"I feel fortunate that my parents always took us on their adventures when they had headache meetings in foreign countries. When I was eight years old—I think that was the first trip—we went to Spain, Portugal, and England. I think we were gone for a month and a half. At least that's what I remember. We went all over Spain, and we went to bullfights, which were pretty wild.

"I remember there was no drinking age, so I think that's when I first experienced wine. Of course, I only had sips of it, but my older sister Judi and I would have a blast. We would drink some wine and, of course, she was older, but I just remember having a really good time and experiencing Europe with her. Those are good memories.

"Then later on, I think when I was ten, we went to Israel and Greece. I'm not positive about the ages, but I'm pretty sure. I had an opportunity to ride a camel, but I discovered I didn't want to ride a camel after all. I got up there, and I started crying. I was pretty scared. And, of course, everyone made fun of me because I wanted to ride the camel, but then I couldn't ride the camel. But he was like perched on this precipice, and I just thought, 'Oh, he's gonna go off the side and I'll die!'

"And then later on when I was seventeen, my parents took me to Italy with them. Again, it was a business trip. I didn't really want to go on that trip because I was seventeen, you know, and I didn't want to go to Europe with my parents. I wanted to stay and hang out with my friends and my boyfriend.

"I had broken my foot prior to the trip, but I healed quickly, and we did wind up having a good time. We went to Venice and I went waterskiing. I got to water-ski on the Adriatic, and it was a lot of fun! I loved waterskiing, so my parents made it worth my while being on that trip."

When the girls were younger, once or twice a year, Seymour would escape the challenge of healing patients and take his family to the Double U, a dude ranch on the outskirts of Tucson, Arizona. There they'd play cowboy/cowgirl for a week or two, riding horses daily, relaxing, and enjoying simple ranch life without telephones or other intrusions of civilization.

The Double U no longer exists today. It was sold and is now known as Canyon Ranch, an upscale health spa. His daughters loved the horses (and were intrigued by the cowboys), so the trip became a Diamond family tradition that provides happy memories even today.

"Originally an old German family ran it," Seymour recalls. "And basically there were two ranches. During those years, there were Jewish ranches and non-Jewish ranches. Really! And there was another one, too, the El Dorado. In complete contrast to the Double U, the El Dorado was very exclusive, not a down-to-earth type ranch.

"We would go out there about twice a year, sometimes once only. There were a group of people who always came out from all over. For example, the owners of Mattel Toys were regulars at the Double U."

Ruth Handler had created the original Barbie doll, and then went on to form Mattel, Inc., with her husband, Elliot, and a partner named Harold Matson. The name Mattel is derived from Matson and Elliot, the names of the male partners.

Mrs. Handler is also known for Nearly Me, a company that produces artificial breasts for women who have been subjected to mastectomy. Her initial motivation for Nearly Me was her own breast cancer diagnosis in 1970 and subsequent mastectomy. The Nearly Me product was designed to be comfortable and natural in appearance, and they were marketed through Neiman Marcus.

"When I conceived Barbie, I believed it was important to a little girl's self-esteem to play with a doll that has breasts," Mrs. Handler once stated. "Now I find it even more important to return that self-esteem to women who have lost theirs."

The Handlers have sinced passed away. They sold Mattell in 1975 following an SEC finding that they'd overstated their earnings.

"I felt it was a wonderful vacation for us to be together, and Elaine felt the same way," Seymour continues about their Double U experience, "although Elaine never rode a horse. I finally persuaded her to give it a try, so she finally got on, rode maybe about ten yards and said, 'I want off!' And off she got. She never wanted to ride again. She sat by the pool, but she never wanted to ride another horse."

The girls, on the other hand, loved it.

"Oh yeah, that was great!" Judi recalls. "We loved it! The family trips were really nice. I thought that was great, the way we always had family trips together. But, yes, the Double U was like a second home. The same families would go back there, year after year. You'd get the same horse and do the same things. It was great!

"And we'd always take the train. I have wonderful memories of that. My father would never fly. I don't know if anybody's told you that. For many, many years he wouldn't fly, so we'd always take the train there. Sometimes we'd go once or twice a year at spring break and Christmas break. I remember loving being in those train cars where you could sleep. In fact, I made Nate once do it with us when our children were little. He hated it.

"I have great memories of the Double U. I think it was really good for my father at the ranch because there was no TV in the rooms, no phone. And our joke with him was—you know, he was always on the phone, he had a phone wherever he was. We had a phone in the bathroom at home! He was always on the phone. But at the ranch, there were no phones or TV.

"He was really into being a cowboy. He had the chaps and the cowboy hat, and he was a different person when he'd get there. It was really relaxing, and it was great!" she concludes.

"I loved the Double U!" Merle exclaims. "It was just fun! We'd go, and my dad would relax, well ... relaxed for him, and my mom really liked it because he didn't have access to a phone. He would ride horses, and we'd be more together as a family."

Amy also has wonderful memories of the Double U. "When I was really young, we'd go twice a year, and that's where I learned to ride horses. I think I was around three years old. Not that I actually remember that, but ... I was quite young.

"I really don't think I had fear of horses because I started so young. And I always wanted to go on the big rides with my sisters and my dad, but it took a while for me to grow old enough to do that.

"They used to make fun of the horses they'd give me. When I first started, I had a horse named Honey. I think every little girl or boy who was riding at the Double U Ranch would ride Honey. I even think my sisters rode Honey. And then later on, they gave me a horse named Deuces, whom I rode for many, many years. Everybody made fun of Deuces, too. They called him an old man, but he was a good horse!

"The ranch was especially fun 'cause they had special events like square dancing, and we played bingo, and it was just a great place. There were families from all over. There were a lot of families from Illinois, too. So I got to be good friends with people and when I would go back, sometimes we would have these little mini-reunions. I made some good friends growing up. I'm not really in touch with anybody now, but it sure was fun!

"I loved the ranch. It was great! There were dogs and horses. And cowboys. As I got older, I really liked the cowboys. I was gonna marry a cowboy. I didn't.

"I really enjoyed that. We had to stop going because they sold the ranch eventually, and we grew up. My sisters stopped going. I think I was around seventeen years old the last year we went. But those are some of my best memories. I just loved the ranch!"

"We had a little shooting range at the ranch," Seymour says, "and I was really a Western buff. In those days, you could carry a gun and nobody stopped you in Arizona. I always was an admirer of Wyatt Earp, so I bought myself a Buntline Special with pearl handles."

According to a popular article written by Jeff Morey that appears repeatedly on the Internet, Wyatt Earp's pistol was produced by Colt's Manufacturing Company as a "revolver-carbine."

But how did the name "Buntline" (which, by the way, reveals no results when searching on Colt's website) become attached to the famous/infamous sidearm?

According to Morey's article, "To fully appreciate the luster history has lent to the 'Special,' its story needs recounting. While an unknown number of extra-long-barreled 'Peacemakers' with standard frames were produced by Colt before World War II, purists reserve the 'Buntline Special' designation for the thirty-one pistols in the serial number range 28,800 to 28,830. The reasoning behind this is that these guns bore special frames that were manufactured for use with oversized barrels in 1876, the very year dime-novelist E. Z. C. Judson—who wrote under the pen name of Ned Buntline—presented an extra-long-barreled Colt .45 to each of five Dodge City lawmen, according to Wyatt Earp's biographer, Stuart Lake. The gifts were allegedly given in gratitude for 'color' the lawmen provided for Buntline's yarns. The recipients were a notable group—Wyatt Earp, Bat Masterson, Bill Tilghman, Charlie Bassett, and Neil Brown. Lake said Masterson and Tilghman found the twelve-inch barrels unwieldy and had them cut down to standard length. Wyatt Kept his 'Special' as received and regarded it his 'favorite over any other gun,' or so Lake tells us."

Or so Lake tells us? Is there room for doubt?

Yes, according to William B. Shillingberg, who apparently did extensive research and presented his findings in an article called "Wyatt Earp and the 'Buntline Special' Myth." The article is long and the complaints are plentiful, but essentially Shillingberg questions the story about Judson/Buntline's presentation of the guns to the lawmen based not on their authenticity, but on the writer's.

Seymour's authenticity, however, is beyond reproach, and so the story continues. "I don't think Wyatt had pearl handles on his, but I wore it around. The ranch also had a skeet shooting area where I enjoyed doing some skeet shooting. I even became quite proficient in hitting skeet with my pistol.

"Everybody used to kid me about carrying my gun, so I said, 'Well, one of these days I'm going to get myself a coyote. There were a lot of coyotes around there. They were howling every night."

Coyotes were a rancher's bane, considered pests, dangerous to livestock, and were frequently killed when the opportunity presented itself, a task typically undertaken by the ranch hands Seymour met at the Double U.

"So, one year, I got myself a coyote whistle that sounded a mating call. I said, 'One of these nights you're going to hear me use it and get my coyote.' Everybody kidded me and finally, the owner's wife, who was a young woman, said to me, 'The day you shoot a coyote, I'm coming out to the pool nude from the waist up.'

"I was out on a ride with one of the cowboys, and I was telling him the coyote story. I asked him, 'How much would it cost for you to get me a coyote?'

"And he said, 'Five bucks.'

"I said, 'Do me a favor. Let me know when you get one. Knock on my cabin door about 10:00 p.m.'

"He agreed, and one afternoon he told me he'd gotten one. So that night, I went around to every cabin and blew my whistle.

Nobody came out, but they knew I was hunting coyote. And about 10:00 p.m. … the ranch hand knocked on my door and said, 'Dr. Diamond, I've got it.'

"I said, 'Bring it out to the corral.'

"He brought the coyote carcass to the corral, and I took out my Buntline Special and shot it twice. I didn't want to lie if anyone asked if I'd really shot it.

"And the next day, everybody was enthralled with the fact that I actually shot a coyote. The woman reneged on the topless bet, but I became a hero to the kids. Everybody came out with their kids. And they started following me around wherever I went."

The Diamonds continued to visit the Double U until it was sold and became Canyon Ranch, a world-class health spa. Merle revisited the ranch in recent years when she and good friend Liz took spent time there to celebrate Merle's fiftieth birthday: "Of course, it's all much different from when we went … all except for the swimming pool area, which looks almost exactly the same. It was funny, but [I] half expected to look up and see Mom sitting beside the pool as she always did during our younger days."

Family vacations took a respite as the kids grew up and spent their time tending to their own families, but the tradition was renewed in 1998 when Elaine and Seymour celebrated their fiftieth wedding anniversary by taking the entire extended family for a Hawaiian vacation. The celebration proved to be so much fun for everyone that the practice continued for six years.

Seymour in trouble with the law? Strange but true. There was an incident involving the Evanston police force, his daughter Amy, and the trampoline she loved.

"Amy was a teenager," Seymour recalls. "I'd bought a professional trampoline for the kids. We had it set up in the backyard, and they all enjoyed it. It was a big one, like the one they use in the circus. They'd used it on *Bozo's Circus*, a television program, for one or two shows. One of the sound engineers at WGN was one of my general practice patients, and he mentioned the trampoline, that they'd bought it to use for a couple shows but now they wanted to get rid of it.

"So I bought the trampoline. We usually kept it folded and locked when it wasn't in use, although not always. It was a menace, a legal menace. One kid broke his arm on it. So I made a rule that nobody could go on it without parental supervision.

"I was out having a dinner with a business partner, not a medical partner, of mine, and I did have a drink or two. Elaine was out with some girlfriends, and Amy was home alone. Amy phoned me and said, 'Dad, these kids are on the trampoline, and I can't get them off.'

"So I said, 'Ask them to get off, tell them they're trespassing, and call the police. I'll come home as soon as I can drive there.' So apparently Amy called the police, and they came. I arrived after the police, and the police shooed them off the trampoline.

"Then the policeman turned and said to me, 'Well, they're just being kids.'

"So I said to him, 'They have no goddamn reason to be on the thing!'

"And he said to me, 'You're swearing in front of a teenager!'

"So I said, 'I don't give a damn what you say; I'm telling you they have no business here!'

"And he said, 'You're under arrest!'

"They took me away in the police car and wanted to book me for swearing in front of a teenager. I didn't even know it was a crime. Then I talked to the sergeant at the station, and he told me that it's *not* a crime! So they had another policeman drive me home. That really bothered me when they took me away like that."

As their daughters ventured on with their careers and marriages, Elaine and Seymour anticipated grandchildren. They weren't disappointed when Judi and Nate led the way.

"Judi and Nate settled in Chicago, and they had their first child, Brian. Elaine and I were in Europe at the time, and Judi was resentful we weren't there. I don't think she ever forgave us. I was getting some honors there.

"Anyway, Brian was born. He was our first grandchild, and we wanted him named religiously. Today, we're not that religious, but back then, there were certain things we wanted. We discussed it with them, but they were in their anti-God phase. They're still in it; they never went out of it. They participate in the social aspects of religion, like a bar mitzvah, but they don't believe.

"I argued with them, that it was a necessity to name him either by a rabbi or at a synagogue. Finally, they said they didn't want it in a house of worship, but I could get a rabbi to do it at their home. But he couldn't mention God.

"I didn't have the courage to go to my own synagogue to ask the rabbi. I just couldn't do it. It would be embarrassing. We found a rabbi who was more liberal. In fact, the other rabbis wouldn't talk to him because he was one of the few rabbis who would marry people even though they had not converted to Judaism. During those times—it's very interesting—it was considered a sin and they ostracized rabbis that did it, and there were only a few that did intermarriage among other more liberal ceremonies.

"So I called him to make an appointment, and I went into his office. I said, 'I've got a problem. I want our first grandchild named religiously, but I don't want you to mention God.'

"I said, 'I'd like you do it at their house.' And so we did it at their house. The rabbi was nice enough; he did a nice naming without mentioning God, and it all worked out."

Brian now lives in Portland, Maine, with his wife, Katie, and their daughter Zevon, Seymour and Elaine's first great-grandchild. Brian and Katie's second child, Oliver James, was born in the spring of 2012. Brian started his career as a financial trader, then studied to become a chef, and now takes care of the kids while his wife, Katie, a medical doctor, tends to her patients.

The Diamond-Falks had a second child, daughter Emily, who lives in Washington, D.C., with her husband, Alex. Both are involved in the world of politics, working for lobbying groups that support their ideals. Emily is communications director at the nonprofit Wilderness Society, and Alex serves as research manager at the Pew Charitable Trust.

Merle and her husband, David (divorced), also brought grandchildren to the Diamond clan, three sons—Max, Michael, and Jacob—and one daughter, Katelynn. And likewise, they're all on their way to becoming successful adults. Max has graduated from the University of Michigan and is, as of 2012, studying law at IIT Chicago-Kent College of Law. Michael also recently graduated from the University of Michigan, and Jacob is pursuing East Asian Studies at Wesleyan University. Katie is a high school student.

Amy decided not to have children. She's the consummate career woman who loves and treats her dogs (Scout and Groovy, her third generation of beloved canines) like two of the world's most spoiled kids.

11. Bridge

"Shortly after Judi was born," Seymour begins, "Elaine would take her out in the carriage. She met some other nice women, and they started talking about taking bridge lessons.

"So we took the lessons and formed a group of about eight couples, and we played what you call social bridge. Social bridge is where you keep score, but it's not a challenging game like duplicate bridge."

According to Wikipedia.com, "Duplicate bridge is the most widely used variation of contract bridge in club and tournament play. It is called *duplicate* because the same bridge deal (i.e. the specific arrangement of the fifty-two cards into the four hands) is played at each table and scoring is based on relative performance. In this way, every hand, whether strong or weak, is played in competition with others playing the identical cards, and the element of skill is heightened while that of chance is reduced. Duplicate bridge stands in contrast to rubber bridge where each hand is freshly dealt and where scores may be more affected by chance in the short run."

"We had no idea about playing duplicate bridge, but one of our pairs was more academic and suggested we try it in our small group. We did it a couple times, and most of the people disliked it because it becomes a competitive game instead of a social game.

"So we just played social bridge for a long time. Then, in about 1956, they had a bridge competition listed in one of the newspapers. It was a citywide Chicago bridge tournament. Elaine and I thought we were pretty good. So we decided it would be fun to enroll in it. And we won the darn thing!

"I had a patient named Jack Taylor, and we became friends with him and his wife. He was one of the premiere early bridge players, and he talked me into playing in a tournament I [had] never played in before, a duplicate tournament.

"He was a literal genius at bridge. You could play out three or four cards, and he could tell everybody what they had in their hands. So it was wonderful playing with him.

"And we won! Not because of me. And this was merely a citywide competition.

"Then I tried to persuade Elaine to try it, but she was very resistant. But they had some local games in Evanston. They had a Friday night game and we would go over and play. A lot of the other players were like Jack Taylor, big-time bridge players.

"And we got beaten badly.

"But we thought we could do better and had little arguments about it, about what we did and what we could do better, and so forth and so on. Bridge was a relatively simple game during those days. They didn't have really complicated systems then. They had some systems, but basic ones. These were the Goren days."

Charles Goren became a world champion bridge player in 1950, having begun to learn the game in the 1920s and then pursuing it with a passion after a girlfriend laughed at his ineptitude at it. He was further inspired by a predecessor bridge expert named Ely Culbertson. Goren's efforts were noticed by Milton Work (who developed the Work Point Count system for playing the game), and Goren began assisting Work with Work's articles and columns. By the mid-1930s, he had published his own book on the game (the first of many to come) called *Winning Bridge Made Easy*.

Elaine, of course, has her own perspective.

"Oh, God," she responded when the subject was brought up. "I enjoyed it after I started it. I was a little concerned about it at first, but then I really enjoyed it. Obviously I'm a competitive person.

"At first I wasn't sure I'd … there are certain rules in duplicate bridge, and I wanted to know that I didn't look foolish doing these rules. We did take lessons, but there are a lot of things to learn, and with each time you play, you learn more. With each lesson you take, you learn more. It really just depends on that. It's a game where you have to think, and you have to count, and you have to remember!

"It's hard. Seymour played with Jim last night because I couldn't go. He's our bridge director at the club, an immensely knowledgeable bridge guy and a very nice person. But Seymour said they had a less than average game. I asked, 'How come?' And he said, 'Jim didn't understand this, and I didn't understand that …' So, even playing with somebody who is a far better player than you are, you can still get it all messed up anyway. It's an understanding between partners. You're actually talking a language.

"You're not going to explain duplicate bridge in this book!" she adds with a laugh.

Nonetheless, bridge soon became a way of life in the Diamond household. Just ask their daughters.

"Do you think it's weird that nobody else in the family plays bridge?" Judi inquires facetiously. "It was obsessive! They would go out and play a few nights a week. It was a very big part of their life."

"I don't know about my sisters," Merle offers, "but I know I had an innate resentment of bridge, and I would never learn how to play it. I always felt like it took my parents away from us. Like 100 percent. I understood they enjoyed it, but they were always playing bridge. I guess the one good thing about it was that when I was in high school, I got to have a ton of parties because they were never at home."

Amy had her own perspective on her parents going out to play bridge in the evening: "They played a lot of it. Still do. I mean, it seems like they play every night. They went out all the time. And as I grew up, that got to be really good because I'd have parties. I'd have big parties!

"My parents would go out and play bridge, and I'd have fifty to a hundred people at my house and get 'em out of the house by the time my parents came home three or four hours later. Yeah, I had great parties. But I think I got that from my sisters because they had parties. Anyway, it was a good opportunity. But, yeah, my parents have been playing bridge forever!"

Seymour continues, "One day, Elaine and I got mixed up in an argument, which you shouldn't do at a bridge table. You know what

I mean. It's not proper. And another couple came over to us, and the man said, 'Why don't you split up? I'll play with your wife and you can play with my wife.'

"They were good players, Ben and Annie Sacks. We would play together from that point, Elaine and I, but we played numerous games with our friends and became very friendly with them. They were much older than we and very proficient. Ben was a bridge teacher as well as a piano teacher, and he gave my girls piano lessons as well. I only have sweet memories of them, and the kids do, too.

"I also became familiar with Al Simons before he came to work for me as our lab technician, and I started to play with him as well as with Elaine. He and I played in a national tournament—I believe the year was around 1960—and I lost my temper at the table. I was playing against some professionals from New York, and I used some swear words I shouldn't have used. And they suspended me for a month! Bridge is supposed to be a gentle person's game. And it really bothered us because we enjoyed the game together, Elaine and I.

"There are various categories that you can attain. Most people want to achieve Life Master status. We achieved Life Master, I believe, in 1962. We started to play as a pair at that time, very rarely with anybody else except for some team games, which we did with other people.

"And we were very successful. At that time, they gave trophies. We threw away about forty of them when we moved. They don't award trophies anymore. Today, it's all about points, whatever you accumulate every year.

"At that time, you needed three hundred to be a Life Master. We are Silver Life Masters right now. There's Life Master Bronze, Silver, Gold, Platinum, and Diamond.

"About 1968, I started to get very involved with the medical practice. We had three daughters, a lot going on. But anyway, we stopped playing. We'd play an occasional game, but not with any frequency, and actually, rarely.

"The time we started back again was about thirty years ago. We had made friends while we were at our winter home in Palm Springs, and we played there. In 1997, they had a regional—that means a whole section of the country was competing. Elaine and I won the most gold. It's a type of point. There are all kinds of points you need and requirements to become a Life Master, but we were past that stage.

"There were about four to five hundred tables there. When we started wintering in Palm Springs, we joined their bridge district. It's an interesting story because we had to speak up to claim our win. We were local members, but people didn't realize it. I had to correct them when they gave it to someone else. I told them, 'I think we did a little better.' They said, 'Well, you're not a member of this unit.' The rule was the trophy went to members who did the best. They assumed we were members in Chicago, which we were not. But once that was straightened out, it was all right.

"But the game was changing. There were specialized conventions, specialized bidding conventions, specialized defensive conventions. Some people you can play against—you don't understand what they're doing! It's not simple.

"I figured if we're going to play, we're going to have to learn some of this new stuff. Basically, we play KIS Bridge. K-I-S. Keep It Simple. And we try our best to keep it simple, but there are some sophisticated things you should learn to keep up and to throw your opponents off. Elaine and I spent a great deal of time learning these.

"There's a resurgence of bridge in places like Florida and Palm Springs because as these people get older, they can't play golf or other more physical activities, so you see a lot of older players. But the younger ones are the sharp ones!

"There are a lot of professionals playing in Palm Springs, which makes it interesting. I mean these people make money out of playing bridge. They charge—and a lot of people can afford it—they charge anywhere from $50 to $400 for playing with somebody.

"There's one man there who has a full-time national player as his partner on a permanent retainer. He pays his expenses and $250,000 a year!

"It's always a pleasure to play against people like that. You lose usually because they really are that good. You can win sometimes, but overall, if you played twenty games against somebody like that, they're going to win more of them.

"One other experience: There are team games where you have four or sometimes six people on a team if you're playing professionally because they change partners.

"We were playing at a large regional in Palm Springs, and who do we draw for the first team we play against? Bill Gates! He didn't have Warren Buffet, but he had three professionals on his team. And he wasn't very chummy, by the way. He's a nerd, really, and we didn't lose too badly. We came pretty close to winning it. But he was playing with three pros, and there were two bodyguards next to him all the way.

"When we returned to bridge after almost a twenty-five-year hiatus, a great number of fancy and difficult systems were in vogue, and we had to incorporate a certain number of them to compete.

"Elaine and I were recently in a team championship game. Naturally, we drew the number one seeded team as our opponents. We sat down at the table, and from the start, we could not understand their bidding and their attitude was arrogant. So I asked them what system they were using and they said, 'The Blue Jay System.'

"I told them we were playing simple bridge, and we beat them sufficiently. As we left the table, I said, 'I guess we played the Eagle System.'

"And that's bridge. It's not simple."

12. Seymour Meets the Mob

Another patient, also introduced on a nighttime house call, would become a good and influential friend, although his career choice provided cause for concern.

"One night, the telephone company gave me a call asking if I could go to see a new patient. It was right in the neighborhood of my office, and the patient was a four-year-old with a severe cough and a fever.

"So I went over to this small apartment, and the father introduced himself as Patrick 'Patsy' Ricciardi. He introduced his wife, and they had two little girls. The younger one had tonsillitis. I examined her and prescribed for her.

"Then he said to me, 'You know, we need a family doctor. We just moved here from the New Jersey area. My cousin does a lot of business in Chicago, and he's bringing me here to help him.'"

"His cousin turned out to be Felix 'Milwaukee Phil' Alderisio, a potent big shot in the mafia. He was an underboss for Salvatore 'Momo' Giancana with credentials as an enforcer, bagman, hit man, and burglar.

"The Ricciardi family kept coming in as my patients, and I could see that they were prospering as time went on. They moved into a house. It was altogether a different mood than when I originally had seen them, and whenever I saw Patsy, he wore a very sharp suit. He was a bail bondsman at the time.

"I always had a nurse working with me, and one day Patsy came into the office with a minor complaint. My nurse wasn't there, so I met him in the reception area.

"'How come you're all alone?' he asked me. I told him my nurse was on jury duty, which was inconvenient.

"'What's her name?' he asked.

"I told him her name," Seymour continued, "and the next day she showed up for work; she'd been released from jury duty. So I knew that I was dealing with a potent character in my friend Patsy."

And that wasn't the only occasion Patsy helped his pal Seymour. In one instance, a disturbed young man whom Seymour had met while treating the man's mother made threatening phone calls, both to Seymour's office and his home.

"I told the police, but they can't do anything until a crime has been committed," Seymour explained. "I really didn't know what else to do, so I told Patsy."

"Patsy said, 'I'll take care of it, so don't worry.'

"I said, 'I don't want anyone to get hurt.'

"And that was the end of it. The guy never bothered us again, and according to his mother, he was alive and well. I guess Patsy was a convincing speaker."

In another story it became apparent that Patsy's persuasive talents weren't limited to threats. He could also be quite charming.

"In about 1977, his wife called to tell me Patsy wasn't feeling well. He was very sick. He had chest pain. The Ricciardis were seeing another doctor at the time because I was specializing in headache by then, but she asked if I would come over and I did.

"She said that he was having severe abdominal pain, but he wasn't. He was really having a coronary artery attack! I hospitalized him at St. Joseph, and I referred him to a cardiologist friend of mine to take care of him.

"I visited him when I made my other rounds. I visited him every day, and on the second day I'm there I saw a woman I didn't recognize as his wife at his bedside. He introduced me to her and said to me, 'She would like to visit me, but not at the same time my wife does.'

"So I talked to the sister in charge of the floor and told her we have a problem. We didn't want to generate another heart attack! So we conveniently arranged a visiting time for everybody. We instructed the wife that she was only allowed these hours, and we told the girlfriend we only wanted her to come the other hours."

Patsy did have a gift for convincing people to see his way. Like the time when Seymour had trouble collecting his share of a real estate sale from a partner.

"Elaine's cousin was a very good lawyer, and during those days, he also bought and sold property as investments. Most of the property was made available in property tax sales. When people didn't pay their taxes, the property was sold to satisfy the tax requirement.

"I was making a good living by then, and Arnie, a lawyer cousin of Elaine's, asked if I would like to invest with him in buying some of these properties. Most of it was vacant land, and I made some money this way.

"One day I bought a lot in Highland Park. It was almost a quarter of an acre, and it was located on a very beautiful street. I thought it was a real bargain when I got it.

"But on the day after I bought it, I got a call from a Mrs. Clavey. Clavey is a famous real estate name; they owned a lot of land in that area. In fact, there's a road called Clavey Road in Highland Park.

"And she said, 'I hope you're happy with my land. I'm glad to be rid of it, because you'll never build on it.' She told me it was fronted on a street where there was a restriction against raising new buildings.

"I called Arnold, and I asked if he had looked it up, and he said, 'Well, you win some, and you lose some.'

"So I paid taxes on it for a couple years. Then I tried to donate it to the city. I thought perhaps they would use it as a little park or something. (They didn't want it, either.)

"The scene now goes to Arizona …

"One year while we were at the Double U Ranch, I was riding horseback, and when we stopped to walk the horses, I struck up a conversation with another guest. I told him I was a doctor, and he told me he was a builder. Not only that, but he lived in Highland Park and did all his building out there.

"So I told him about this lot, and he said, 'Well, let's have our lawyers draw up some papers, and we'll get a house built!'

"He said, 'There's a law that says they can't stop you if you get your construction project under a roof. I'll do it over the Labor Day weekend. We'll start Friday afternoon, and by the time the building inspectors come back to work the following Tuesday, we'll have a roof on it.'

"So, I made the deal, and we were going to split the profit on the house. The house was built, and it was sold. Three months went by, and I kept calling the builder asking him for my share, but he kept stalling me.

"So, I'm on the phone and I'm yelling. It was at the office. I had evening hours, and I'm yelling at my lawyer. I said, 'Why can't you do something about it?'

"Well, Patsy happened to be in the office at the time, and he asked, 'Who is exciting you, Dr. Diamond?' And I told him the story.

"He said, 'Do you mind if I talk to him?'

"I said, 'No, I don't mind, but I don't want to wish anybody any harm.'

"Two days went by, and I received a phone call at about 4:00 p.m. It was the builder! He said, 'Seymour, I've got to see you. Tonight.'

"I said, 'Well, you know, you owe me money.'

"He said, 'I want to settle up with you.'

"He came to my office and met me at about 6:00 p.m., and he paid me what he owed me in cash, $100 bills. And then he says to me, 'I know you waited. Do I owe you any interest?'" Patsy evidently had covered all possibilities in his discussion with the builder.

Early in Seymour's phase as a general practitioner, he brought another doctor into the office, an East Coast physician. Seymour was also working on an exhibit for the pharmaceutical company Lederle at the time, and he enlisted this doctor to help in doing the research and putting the exhibit together.

"I did this exhibit on hypertension for Lederle," Seymour said. "I presented it at some major meetings, and it won a couple of prizes, ribbons, medals, etc., and I also published an article on the work.

"About six months after I first published the article, I received a letter from a physician. It came to me because I was the major publisher of the article. He claimed that we had stolen his illustrations demonstrating hypertension, and we did not give him any acknowledgement, which is a no-no. I explained that I was unaware that this was not original work and apologized. Then I had some very stern words with the doctor working in my office about ethics. Apparently he'd stolen many ideas from somebody else's work without asking their permission to use it. It's not a copyright violation, but it was unethical.

"Another six months went by after this episode, and I became aware that this doctor was having an improper relationship in my office with a woman who was married to a dentist friend of mine. She was originally a patient of mine. She came in once when I wasn't there, and he saw her, and they developed an improper relationship. She was a married woman with kids.

"When I found out about it, I dismissed him from my staff. This was two strikes, and I don't wait for the third strike.

"Another three months went by, and this doctor subsequently separated from his wife. He had a brother-in-law who ran a pharmacy near my office on Western Avenue. I had no relationship with this man, except that I was a busy practitioner and he incidentally filled a number of my patients' prescriptions.

"But then I got a call from him and he said to me, 'Dr. Diamond, I'd like to talk to you. It's very important.' And I said to him, 'What is so important?' And he said, 'It's a matter of life and death.' So I said, 'Come on in and we'll talk.'

"He came into my office, and I asked him what was wrong. He replied, 'I know you dismissed my former brother-in-law. And before he separated from his wife, my sister, he asked me if I knew anybody that could act as a hit man against you!'

"He felt obligated to warn me. So, I called the police and went over to the station and talked with them about it. But they said, 'Well, unless you have some proof, we can't do anything about it. It may be just hearsay.' The police didn't want to do anything. And in the meantime, through another channel, I heard a second time that this doctor was making inquiries about a hit man.

"With the lack of interest from the police force, I decided that I would call my friend Patsy Ricciardi. Once again, he said he would talk to whoever was bothering me, and that I should never worry again. He didn't hurt the doctor, of course, but he talked to him. And that was the end of it."

Then Seymour describes an unusual visit from Patsy in June 1985.

"He came in to say hello to me and asked what he should do about certain bruises he had on his face and body. Big bruises. I asked, 'Is everything all right?' He reassured me. I examined him. I told him the bruises would heal all right by themselves. He was really black and blue, but he wouldn't tell me how it happened."

Despite Patsy Ricciardi's lifestyle, which certainly included a fair share of crime and violence, he remained a good friend to Seymour until the day he died.

Selected excerpts from the *Chicago Tribune*, July 27, 1985:

Missing Porn-Theater Owner Found Dead In Car Trunk

When a body identified as that of Patrick Ricciardi, minor crime syndicate figure and owner of a porn movie house, was found in the trunk of a car on the North Side Friday, authorities were certain the death was mob related.

But they said they have no idea why Ricciardi, 59, was killed.

When it was reported that the victim's trouser pockets had been turned inside out and that as much as $1,000 was missing, some speculated Ricciardi may have owed money to his killers.

Ricciardi vanished Wednesday after telling a daughter he was going to a meeting with an unidentified person at Halsted and Webster Streets.

The body, with bullet wounds in the back and head, was identified as Ricciardi by Frank Oliver, his lawyer and one-time business partner.

Police found the body Friday when they pried open the trunk of a stolen 1980 Oldsmobile that had been abandoned under a railroad viaduct at 1651 W. Webster St. The car was parked a mile west of where Ricciardi's meeting was to have taken place.

Police said Ricciardi may have been expecting trouble at his appointment. Although his late-model Lincoln sedan was parked outside at the time, he phoned his daughter from the Admiral Theater Wednesday morning and asked her to drive him to the meeting.

The daughter told police that she declined and he said he would go by cab.

Oliver told a reporter that Ricciardi was never connected to the mob and speculated that robbery might have been the motive for his killing.

"I read his obituary in the paper, and then his wife called to tell me that he had died," Seymour recalls. "I asked her to let me know about his funeral arrangements. I certainly had respect for him as a person because of the way he treated me. Not as a gangster, but as a person.

"They were having a wake for him, she said, and she gave me the name of the funeral parlor. It was one of the large funeral parlors on Harlem Avenue in Chicago. I asked Elaine's sister Barbara and her husband, Hank, if they'd like to go to dinner with us near the funeral home; it was in an Italian neighborhood. And then they could wait in the car while I made a condolence call.

"I parked the car two blocks away. I figured they were going to be checking license plates to see who was going in and out. So I walked the two blocks, and I went into the funeral home.

"They had a bulletin board that listed which visitation room people were in. But I didn't see the name Patrick Ricciardi. It wasn't there. So I went into the main office and said, 'I'm looking for the wake of Patrick Ricciardi. Where is the visitation room?'

"And he said to me, 'It's on the lower level.'

"I went down there, and there was his wife, his two kids, a closed casket, and nobody else. I was the only one, other than his family, who attended Patsy's wake.

"The only one," Seymour repeats. "Isn't that tragic?"

13. Neurology Beckons

"When we returned to Chicago," Seymour recalls, "I wanted to get experience in neurology. I needed to make a living, so I maintained my family practice, but I still wanted to do neurology.

"So I went to see the head of the neurology department at Chicago Medical School, where I graduated—Harry Garner, a very nice man. I went to visit him at the school and told him about my interest in neurology. So he set up a preceptorship for me. He didn't charge me. He was very magnanimous about it."

A preceptorship occurs when the preceptor, a practicing physician, gives personal instruction, training, and supervision to another physician.

"During those years, they established various boards; there was a neurology board and a psychiatric board. Under the preceptorship, I would never be eligible to take the neurology board exam—I would have had to devote two or three years as a resident at a hospital doing neurology, and I didn't want to do that at this time. So the preceptorship took its place.

"We met about every two weeks, and he tested me and taught me. After about year of this preceptorship, he said, 'I'd like you to be a clinical assistant at the medical school.' He gave me a medical school appointment in the Department of Neurology. Clinical assistant, which is the lowest appointment you can get.

"He was attending at Cook County Hospital and at the Oak Forest Infirmary. As part of my duties, I made rounds with him at both institutions. I did the rounds when he could not do them, and ultimately I became an attending physician in neurology at the Cook County Hospital and Oak Forest Infirmary. I eventually became adjunct associate professor in neurology at Chicago Medical School and professor in the Department of Pharmacology at the same school.

"I never was a board-approved neurology physician. I never could take the exam. But you don't have to be board-approved for the American Medical Association to list you as whatever specialty you want to be in. So, I'm listed as a neurologist with the AMA, and I consider myself to be a neurologist. And such was my progression into neurology before the headache work."

Seymour was a board-approved family practice doctor, and he was also head of the family practice section at both Illinois Masonic Hospital and St. Joseph Hospital.

"During the time I was head of the family practice at St. Joseph, I was instrumental in the hospital's getting an approved residency in family practice, which was difficult to do in those years.

"I also helped form the DePaul Family Clinic. It was one of the first outpatient clinics formed specifically to serve the poor. Elaine also volunteered a lot of her time to help with the social work it took to get this clinic started."

Detail men, as they're called, are representatives of the pharmaceutical companies who call on doctors to introduce them to the companies' new products and encourage their use.

One such detail man, Randy Barth, who represented the pharmaceutical company Merck, came to call on Seymour with a request.

"He asked if I would be interested in doing some research with them," Seymour remembers. "I said I'd like to learn more about it, so he had Dr. Clyde Strickland contact me. We had dinner and discussed the opportunity.

"And by the way, this is the turning point in my life."

Dr. Strickland told Seymour that Merck was working on a new type of antidepressant and explained the pharmacology of the new drugs to him. Up to this time, the only antidepressants available were MAO inhibitors, and although they are effective, there are risks associated with their use.

"Basically, these drugs work on the neurotransmitters to neutralize depression," Seymour explains. "These MAO inhibitors, however, interreacted with certain foods and drugs. If doctors and their patients weren't careful about the patient's diet, the patient could have an extreme hypertension episode (high blood pressure). They'd be going up to 260, 280, and possibly stroke. So they had to be very careful about their diet and other medicines!

"Dr. Strickland told me about this new group of drugs, and that they work. They're called tricyclics. A psychiatrist in Baltimore by the name of Frank Ayd had published preliminary research about their use in depression. He also mentioned that a neurologist from Australia, Dr. James Lance, had used tricyclics with success on a patient or two with headache. He noted that even in nonobviously depressed patients who had somatic physical complaints—arthritis, chronic fatigue, all those kinds of symptoms—or minimally depressed that wasn't obvious; they exhibited physical, medical, and mental manifestations, which you wouldn't relate to depression.

"Dr. Strickland wanted to know if I would do a project with some of my patients, with their permission, to see how they responded. Specifically, he wanted to know more about how the tricyclics worked with patients who had physical complaints and were only minimally depressed, not depressed enough to see a psychiatrist or to get any of that sort of treatment.

"I agreed to do a study with a limited number of patients. It was what we call an open label study. Nowadays, you have to test a drug against a placebo, and the study has to be a lot more rigid in the criteria. I had a fantastic response from a large group of patients.

"Dr. Strickland came in, and I went over the study results with him. He liked what he saw and asked if I would like to present something about this research in the form of an exhibit. Nowadays, people who present do it either at a formal talk at a meeting or they prepare posters, just a large board displaying their research.

"Exhibits were large, usually sixteen feet compared with a poster, which would be four or five feet. And they were produced by graphic arts professionals. Robert Thompson was our designer, and we produced a very elaborate exhibit called Masks of Depression.

"The exhibit didn't mention Merck's specific tricyclic product. If I'd advertised their brand name, I'd have been disqualified. I used the generic classification of the drugs, talked about the improvement in my patients, and showed the figures that documented the improvement."

Seymour's exhibit was on display at the 1961 American Medical Association meeting in Atlantic City, and he was also on-site explaining it to interested parties. It was there that he was approached by a doctor from Washington, D.C., Lester Blumenthal, who asked a fateful question:

Have you ever tried tricyclics on headache patients?

"He left me his card," Seymour said, "And he said, 'If you ever do any work in headache, let me know. I would be very interested.'

"He was an internist who, with his partner, saw a fair number of headache patients but was not doing research. So it set off a little light in me. I thought it would be interesting.

"I was extremely enthusiastic about this, so I discussed it with Dr. Strickland, and he set up a study for me through Merck on a protocol, as they call it, to study a group of patients who were marginally depressed and for whom headache was one of their symptoms.

"Let me qualify it to say that some of these were migraines. Some of these were what we call mixed headache or chronic migraine. Some of them had what we call tension headache. I was not supposed to differentiate at this point.

"I put together a group—I think we tested about sixty patients over a year or a year and a half. Clinically, the same trial would never be accepted today, but I became fascinated. I knew the drug worked on a good portion of headache patients.

"At the time I thought all these people had a hidden or masked depression. I called Dr. Blumenthal one day, and he asked me if I'd like to present my findings to his organization, the American Association for the Study of Headache (AASH). It had about maybe thirty to thirty-five members who were very diverse in specialties. I would say practically none of them were neurologists."

Dr. Blumenthal was one of the founders of AASH, and the group was about three years old at the time. They'd planned a meeting in conjunction with the American Medical Association in San Diego, California.

"A lot of the specialty societies had meetings in conjunction with the AMA back then. Dr. Blumenthal asked if I would like to present my work. I accepted and presented the results of my work, which I referred to as depressive headache. Later on, I learned that this group of drugs has inherent properties against pain itself in addition to depression. But at that time I presented the paper, I talked about depression and headache. My work with the tricyclic antidepressants initiated their use as the primary treatment for chronic headache. They are still one of the most prescribed drugs for that indication.

"There were some very important people in medicine in general at this meeting for the American Association for the Study of Headache. Among them was Bayard Horton, who was a very famous clinician from the Mayo Clinic. Also attending was Walter Alvarez, one of the most famous clinicians at the Mayo Clinic, primarily with GI diseases, but a very famous man. I was really impressed!"

Dr. Bayard T. Horton was one of the original pioneers of headache study. After studying medicine and gaining his B.S. and M.D. degrees in Virginia, Horton continued his education at the University of Minnesota, where he earned his M.S. degree in medicine. He then worked at the Mayo Clinic, and over a twenty-year period, he examined more than 1,400 headache patients. Cluster headaches, the ones nicknamed "suicide headaches" due to their severity and the patient's willingness to do literally anything to halt the pain, were originally called Horton's cephalalgia because Bayard Horton offered the first theory about their cause. He contributed numerous papers and lectures on headache, and in 1974 was awarded the Distinguished Clinician Award by the American Association for the Study of Headache.

In 1926, a year after Seymour was born, Dr. Walter C. Alvarez joined the Mayo Clinic as a consultant in internal medicine, and during his tenure there, he researched and generated nearly 350 scientific articles. Most of his work dealt with the digestive tract and its associated diseases and neuroses. Working with associate George Little, Dr. Alvarez constructed a motion picture X-ray machine, and with it he observed the movement of the digestive tract in action. He completed, in collaboration with Dr. Cesare Gianturco, a study of the emptying of the stomach and another on the behavior of the pylorus (the section of the stomach that connects to the duodenum). Even after his retirement in 1950, he continued writing books as well as a syndicated medical column that reached twelve million readers.

It was also at this AASH meeting that Seymour would meet another presenter named Donald Dalessio. Dr. Dalessio would become a good friend, and later in their careers, they would publish medical books together.

"There were a number of papers presented at the meeting, but nobody presented anything similar to what I talked about. They had a little gathering afterward. There weren't a lot of people at the meeting, so there weren't many who went to this social gathering afterward. I got along socially with Dr. Blumenthal and an internist by the name of Perry McNeal. We sat there and talked around the table."

Little did Seymour know then that he'd soon become an integral part of this new headache organization.

"I went back to Chicago, and about a week or two later, Dr. Blumenthal called me and said that there had been some discord between groups within the organization. 'This is a small organization to have discord,' he said, 'and you seem like a very amiable person.' Then he asked if I would become secretary of the American Association for the Study of Headache. The secretary's duties were to line up meetings, to communicate with the members, doing the programs, inviting the people …

"Suddenly, I was in charge of the whole thing! It was like running the organization. And at the same time, Dr. Dalessio became editor of the organization's journal."

Seymour had become secretary of AASH in 1965. He was promoted several times, becoming executive secretary in 1971 and ultimately accepting the title of executive director, an office he'd hold from 1976 through 1985. Under his guidance, the group would grow in size from around one hundred members to more than 550.

At about the same time Seymour began working with AASH, the American Medical Association had special groups, a precursor to what would become medical specialties. One of the groups dealt with neurology and at the time was combined with psychiatry. But within the neurology group, there was a headache subdivision in which all the members were neurologists except one: John Graham. Seymour was not a member.

"The headache group ran a small scientific meeting—maybe six to eight people—by invitation only, so I couldn't go to it. It was run by a person who later became my friend, Arnold Friedman, one of the pioneers in headache treatment and research."

During his tenure with AASH, Seymour was instrumental in recruiting innovative and influential doctors into the association, among them Dr. John Graham and Dr. Arnold Friedman.

Dr. John Ruskin Graham had received his education at Harvard Medical School, graduating in 1934. He then joined a group of physicians who were operating one of the first clinics to treat headache patients at Massachusetts General Hospital. He went to New York for a year to do research with Dr. Harold G. Wolff. Other accomplishments include teaching at Harvard Medical School as well as at Tufts University School of Medicine. He was chief of medical services at Boston's Faulkner Hospital from 1950 to 1974, where he also founded the Headache Research Foundation in 1950.

At Faulkner, Graham found various innovative ways to treat headache, including corticosteroids and an ergotamine-caffeine suppository for the treatment of migraine headaches. He also noted the side effects of the headache medicine Sansert and oversaw beta-blocker and lithium studies. He received the Menninger Award in 1982, given by the American College of Physicians for his contributions to mental health.

Seymour recalls, "It was a real breakthrough that I was able to encourage him to become a member. One of the other internists, Perry McNeal, who was an officer at that time, helped me with it. It was considered a coup because having a member with Dr. Graham's credentials bolstered our young organization's credibility."

Dr. Arnold P. Friedman proved to be more difficult to recruit. He was well established as an expert in headache treatment, having founded the United States's first hospital-based headache clinic at the Montefiore Medical Center in the Bronx in the mid-1940s. The Swiss pharmaceutical company Sandoz (now Novartis) sponsored the clinic in its early years and, in fact, named one of its products after the clinic: Fiorinal, a combination of aspirin, butalbital (more commonly known as phenobarbital), and caffeine.

"Still, Dr. Friedman remained aloof from us," Seymour relates. "And I never really had any contact with him. I had contact with one of his associates, Dr. Arthur Elkind, who was one of the people who helped Dr. Friedman in the charity clinic he ran at Montefiore Medical Center.

"I had met Dr. Elkind when I was doing my exhibits on headache; he was doing one for Friedman. He was a very amiable person, and he told me how resistant Dr. Friedman was to our organization. Dr. Elkind told me that it wouldn't do any good if I approached him or not, and I took it on face value.

"During that time, I was at our Tarpon Springs meeting, and John Edmeads, a neurologist from Toronto, had written some papers, although he wasn't presenting a paper at our meeting. I encouraged him to join our organization. He was the only one I knew from Canada who had attained some stature in headache medicine. Subsequently we became friends, and John served as president of the AHS from 1982 through 1984.

"I was doing a lot of speaking, and at that time, there was a headache clinic at Mount Sinai Hospital in New York. It was run by Dr. David Coddon. He was a neurologist, a very nice person, but a little unconventional in his ideas.

"He's also famous for an incident that involved a suicide jumper, his headache treatment, and a shooting in New York City. A young heiress jumped from a multistory building, committing suicide. An Iranian immigrant, here in the U.S. to study acting, was hit in the head by the falling heiress and subsequently developed a headache problem.

"The Iranian went to Dr. Coddon and received the doctor's treatment for several years. In the meantime, Dr. Coddon was also called upon to testify in the Iranian's lawsuit against the heiress' estate, a process that typically involves payment for the time one spends in court.

"When the legalities were finally settled, however, Coddon hadn't been fully paid for his medical or his legal services, and of course, he approached the Iranian about his payment.

"But the Iranian thought he'd been overbilled, and he threatened to sue Dr. Coddon unless the bill amount was lowered. Dr. Coddon refused to change his billing.

"So then the Iranian called Dr. Coddon at his office, cursed him, and said he was going to come over and kill the doctor. Dr. Coddon locked himself in the library at his office and retrieved a handgun, which he was licensed to carry in New Jersey where he lived.

"The Iranian arrived brandishing a gun, kicked down the library door, and was shot by Dr. Coddon! Fortunately, the bullet didn't kill him, and he was arrested soon thereafter, but so was Dr. Coddon. Although he was licensed to carry the firearm in New Jersey, his office was in New York. The Iranian went to jail, and Dr. Coddon paid a fine for his gun-toting infraction.

"Later, Dr. Coddon decided to run a daylong headache seminar in New York City. He invited me to be one of his guest speakers, and another speaker was Arnold Friedman. It happened that we were sitting close to each other at this meeting. I presented my work, and Dr. Friedman presented his work.

"Toward the end of the meeting, Dr. Coddon presented what he called the 'Coddon Cocktail.' It contained three effective medicines in the prevention of migraine, but one would not use them in combination as a first treatment. One might want to combine one or two at some later date, but the idea of using them as a starting regime was probably inappropriate. When Dr. Coddon had completed his talk—and his was the final talk of the day—Dr. Friedman looked at me and shook his head, and I looked at him and I shook my head. And we started to talk.

"I said, 'Would you like to have a drink?' And he said, 'Well, I don't drink, but I'll go out and have some tea with you someplace.' We went into one of the restaurants, I had some coffee, he had some tea, and we started to talk. And at that time, he was contemplating leaving his private practice, giving up his clinic at Montefiore Medical Center, and moving to Arizona

"I told him that we had a large membership and that I would be very honored if he would join us. I more or less had control of nominating committees at that time. I assured him that I would have him start, and within a year he would be vice president, and within two years he would be president. We negotiated, and he joined our organization.

"As when we recruited Dr. Graham, it was a big coup for the organization because it resulted in a great number of other practitioners, primarily neurologists, joining the organization. We also got some financial support for the association from Sandoz through our relationship with Dr. Friedman."

Not all ran smoothly when Dr. Friedman became a member and rose to the office of president. It was his intent to improve the standards of the organization and of its journal publication. In expressing his concerns, Dr. Friedman precipitated confrontations with the society's treasurer, Dr. Robert Ryan, and its journal editor, Dr. Lee Kudrow, who by then had replaced Dr. Dalessio.

Dr. Friedman was particularly critical of the journal, its selection of journal articles, how they were selected, how they were edited—nothing seemed to be good enough. As a result, Dr. Kudrow wrote a letter tending his resignation as editor due to Dr. Friedman's actions, although he remained a member of the society. Dr. John Edmeads assumed the editorship position.

"He was not an easy man to get along with, although we were fine," Seymour recalls of Dr. Friedman. "He was a very pompous little man. But I got along with a lot of pompous little people, and we later developed a firm relationship."

Like a medical practice, once a foundation is formed, it must grow. How much it grows depends on many factors, but among the positive ones is finding and working with other good people.

"At one of my earlier meetings with the AASH, I met a very interesting Danish physician, Torvald Dalsgaard-Nielsen, who practiced neurology but also enjoyed working with headache. He gave a talk at one of our meetings, and then he and I discussed the idea of running an international meeting. We planned it for Elsinore, Denmark, in May of 1971. He publicized it in Europe while we publicized it in the United States.

"One of the fascinating things about it was trying to get a charter plane to take everybody over from here. I called various airlines, and they came in to talk to me. Finally TWA came in, the old Trans World Airlines, and they offered a six-day stay in Denmark. We paid for our own hotels there because they didn't fly into Denmark. That wasn't their usual route.

"They offered me a 707 that seated about 145 people to fly from Chicago, land in New York, pick up New York passengers, fly to Denmark, wait for us for five or six days—whatever it was—and then fly us all back. And I booked it for $27,500!

"The trip was very successful. From a personal aspect, I met many of my Scandinavian and other European colleagues who were doing headache work, and it became, from my own career point of view, a very significant event. A book of all the papers was published, and I was the coeditor with Dr. Nielsen. It was very good for my career."

Later, when traveling in Europe, Seymour learned that Dr. Dalsgaard-Nielsen was dying of cancer. He rescheduled his appointments and took an extra day to go to Denmark to visit his friend. It was a "good visit," he recalls, and he was grateful for the opportunity to say goodbye.

Another influential headache pioneer was Dr. Harold Wolff; he was named the first occupant of the "Anne Parrish Titzel Chair" for the Department of Internal Medicine and Neurology at Cornell University.

"During my early years as I ascended and started to work in headache, after I had left general practice, I was influenced by—probably more so than Arnold Friedman—a researcher in headache named Harold Wolff. I don't think he saw many patients, but he did some very basic research in headache, and some of his basic research still stands today. He did a lot of his work with his research assistant, Helen Goodell."

Among the accomplishments of the Wolff/Goodell partnership (in this case, in association with Dr. James D. Hardy in 1940) is the invention of a dolorimeter, a device to measure the level of pain. With it, they developed a scale called the Hardy-Wolff-Goodell scale that designated 10 pain levels called "dols." Obviously, subjecting human test patients to pain seems controversial by today's standards, although at that time, similar and even more worrisome experiments were taking place.

Even a quick Internet search will reveal that experiments we'd consider unspeakable today were performed throughout the history of medicine, and while they were often brutal—even to the point of killing the subjects after painful experiments—they did provide a knowledge base that's useful in contemporary treatment.

In 1954, for example, Dr. Wolff was involved in a CIA project called QKHILLTOP to study Chinese brainwashing techniques and then create a new system the CIA might use in their own interrogations. Wolff requested information from the CIA about "threats, coercion, imprisonment, deprivation, humiliation, torture, 'brainwashing,' 'black psychiatry,' and hypnosis, or any combination of these, with or without chemical agents."

And in return, his research team would then "assemble, collate, analyze, and assimilate this information and will then undertake experimental investigations designed to develop new techniques of offensive/defensive intelligence use. . . . Potentially useful secret drugs (and various brain damaging procedures) will be similarly tested in order to ascertain the fundamental effect upon human brain function and upon the subject's mood. . . . Where any of the studies involve potential harm of the subject, we expect the Agency to make available suitable subjects and a proper place for the performance of the necessary experiments," according to Wolff.[1]

Similar standards were applied in headache research on human test subjects.

"He would do craniotomies [open the skull to view the brain] in various stages of migraine attacks," Seymour states, bringing Wolff's story back to the subject of headache treatment. "His work talks about the beginning of the headache where you have the aura, the warning of headache where the blood vessels constrict. And then, once the headache occurs after the warning, the blood vessels on that side of the brain dilated or expanded. And while they expanded, they appeared to be inflamed.

"Most inflammation is caused by infection—germs—but Dr. Wolff described the inflammation that appeared in patients with prolonged attacks as 'sterile.' He also analyzed the inflammation to make sure of what was happening.

"He wrote *Wolff's Headache and Other Head Pain*, the standard text on headache. Nobody had written a book like this, based on his research. And despite any controversy, the results of his research became very useful.

---

[1] Source: www.4thmedia.org

"He was so egotistical and sure of himself, according to conversations with many of my colleagues, that he never took the board examinations for either neurology or medicine," Seymour adds. "He said that he didn't think the people giving him the exam were capable of examining him. He did some experiments in the 1950s that today would be found unacceptable by any ethical hospital review committee on research. They'd probably remove him from the staff. But it took somebody of his nature to do these things."

Ironically, Dr. Wolff died in 1962 of cerebral vascular disease, killed by the very blood vessels he studied. Dr. Wolff's research was the most important work in headache during the twentieth century.

"He was the man!" Seymour emphasizes. "I invited his widow to become an honorary member of our organization, and she went along with us when we went over to Europe. Helen Goodell also joined us on the trip, which was wonderful."

"Artist Isabel Bishop was Dr. Wolff's widow. I have one of her drawings at our Palm Springs house," he continues. "She became a very close friend of Elaine's and mine. When we went to New York, we usually invited her to dinner, but she insisted on taking us to her club because she didn't want us to pay.

"She took us to her studio one day, and it was in the same building as Andy Warhol's studio, The Factory, at 33 Union Square West. She took us to his studio and introduced us. It was in the Decker Building, a Manhattan landmark.

"The only other anecdote I have is that, when she died, she had almost a whole page obit in the *New York Times*. Dr. Wolff got only about a quarter of a page for his obituary, and I think he probably turned over in his grave! She was a very sweet woman."

In 1972, *Good Housekeeping* magazine printed an article about Seymour's headache work titled "Head Hunters," written by William Barry Furlong. Soon thereafter, Seymour received a call from a literary agent in New York, who asked if he'd be willing to write a book. At the time, he was extremely busy building his new headache practice and speaking at medical meetings, so he told the agent he simply didn't have time.

That didn't stop the agent. He contacted the writer William Barry Furlong, located a publisher who was willing to take on the project, and introduced Seymour to Furlong. In preparation for the new book, which would be called *More Than Two Aspirin*, Furlong spent six weeks with Seymour at his clinic. With the patients' permission, Furlong accompanied Seymour through his entire day's work, and the final manuscript presented twenty-five separate types of headache patients, their disorders, and treatments. It was written in easily understood terms so that any reader could gain an understanding of headache treatment.

When published in 1976, the book was the first comprehensive layperson's book about headache. It was distributed worldwide and had a powerful effect on establishing Seymour as a headache expert.

At the time, Furlong and Seymour argued about the book's title, with Seymour ultimately getting his way despite Furlong's determination to name the book *Hope for Your Headache Problem*. In retrospect, Seymour admits that Furlong was probably right, and in its revised edition, published in 1988 with Seymour's journalist daughter Amy, the title became *Hope for Your Headache Problem—More Than Two Aspirin*.

Promoting the book in typical fashion (radio, TV, book signings), Seymour went on several book tours, which he found frustrating. Despite having a driver to spirit him from interview to interview, the schedule called for ten to twelve stops every day, and in some instances, the locations didn't even have the book in stock. He recalls the experience as hectic and laughingly states that he doesn't want to do it again.

Another project that helped establish the Diamond Headache Clinic was a book written by Seymour and an associate, Dr. Donald Dalessio, called *The Practicing Physician's Guide to Headache*.

"Up until the time we wrote that book, the only books on headache study were highly technical, nonclinical, and oriented toward research rather than practical application," Seymour explains.

Dr. Harold G. Wolff had written *Headache and Other Head Pain* based on his extensive research. That tome was in its second edition when the Diamond/Dalessio book was written in 1972.

Seymour admired Dr. Wolff's work, but found that it didn't include practical treatment information to help physicians treat patients.

"It was so nonclinical and oriented towards research," he said, "that it became useless for any practicing physician to gain any knowledge of how to actually treat the patient."

Seymour quotes from the book's preface: "It is not the purpose of this book to be a reference text, giving a multitude of information. Rather, we hope to demonstrate a definitive approach to both the diagnosis and treatment of headaches. An attempt has been made to keep the text uncluttered, simple, and easy to follow.

"Two important factors are paramount in the treatment and management of headache patients. The first is that perhaps half of them have been treated symptomatically without regard to a diagnosis, and with drugs used simply to relieve pain. There should be a logical sequence employed in investigating the problem. Many headache patients have not had a careful history or neurological examination, nor has an adequate attempt been made to diagnose the type of headache from which they suffer.

"Even though the history and neurological examinations are keys to the diagnosis, extensive testing procedures may have been performed without discrimination. It was the ardent intention to promote and provide a logical understanding of headache patients and be coached to diagnosis and treatment of his or her problem.

"To the patient who has suffered over a long period of time, his headache is most important, not 'just a headache'. He or she will travel from doctor to doctor, and to large research and diagnostic centers. This brings us to our second important point: Diagnosis must be coordinated with continual treatment.

"The headache patient needs attention and treatment on a continuing basis, whether the diagnosis indicates psychological, vascular, or organic causes. The follow-up treatment may be on the basis of trial and error, until relief is afforded.

"I'd like to add something here," he says, pausing in his reading of the preface. "Sometimes I see a patient I can't help. They've been in, and we've tried everything without success. I once asked one of the patients, 'Why are you still coming to see me?' And he said, 'You're the only one that cares.'

He continues to read: "The patient must have full confidence in his physician and the physician's approach to the problem. It's easier for one physician to mold this confidence than sending them to a series of consultants.

"Another principle in writing the book was that we said physicians should not be intolerant of their headache sufferer. It's easy to lose patience and lack concern for these people, especially those with persistent complaints. The simplest course by many doctors is to blame the problem on a defective personality, or the wish of their patient to avoid reality. Careful attention to symptoms and related details, however, will often reveal the cause and guide the subsequent treatment."

Medcom Press published *The Practicing Physician's Approach to Headache* in 1973. They changed publishers in 1977, going this time with Williams & Wilkins for the second edition.

"Then in 1990, the sixth—and final—edition was published," Seymour adds.

"Dr. Dalessio and I decided that that was enough of this book. We had nurtured it, but we didn't feel we wanted to rewrite it again. We gave it to a couple of young physicians who were supposed to continue with it. But they never followed through, except with the sixth edition, but never followed through after that."

The Physician's Approach to Headache became one of the most popular books of its time. Several pharmaceutical companies purchased the book in bulk quantities and shared them with their physician customers, often with Seymour in attendance for a book-signing event. It was published in Italian and Spanish versions and distributed worldwide, helping educate doctors in headache treatment while further enhancing the Diamond Headache Clinic's credibility.

As Seymour became more and more interested in pursuing headache as a specialty, he found he'd have to leave another associate behind.

"Up until 1974, I still had my general practice, and I was seeing a lot of headache patients. I had a partner at that time, Dr. Bernard Baltes, a very nice man. He was a Ph.D. as well as an M.D. I took him into the practice, and he was with me for almost seven years. He had worked previously for industry and had at one time a senior position with Riker Pharmaceuticals. They're not in existence today. We were friends because of some of the research I did for his company. But when I decided to specialize in headache, he wanted to continue with the general medicine, so we separated."

And thus, through his association with other pioneers of headache medicine, Seymour opened his Diamond Headache Clinic in 1974. It was the first private headache clinic in the world, an unproven concept in the world of medicine at the time, and as such, a courageous decision on Seymour's part. Other headache clinics had been included within hospitals' specialty departments, but no one until now had opened a practicing doctor's office to serve only people who suffered from head pain.

14. Diamond Headache Clinic

E ven as he opened the one-of-a-kind medical clinic that would become his legacy, a deep sadness enveloped Seymour on August 13, 1974, when his father died. The *Chicago Tribune* printed this basic obituary the day after.

> Nathan Diamond, 81, retired agent for the Metropolitan Life Insurance, Co. died yesterday in his home at 2720 West Glenlake Avenue. He retired in 1964 after fifty years with the company. Survivors include his widow, Rose; two sons, Dr. Seymour and Dr. Alfred; two daughters, Ann and Mrs. Idell Applebaum; and nine grandchildren.

"We always had a close relationship," Seymour recalls. "He would very often visit me at the office when he knew I had some time off. We'd talk about family and things. I really miss him for that.

"When he was diagnosed with his lung cancer, no matter how busy I was, I personally brought him in for each treatment at the hospital. He underwent radiation treatment, and I made sure I was the one who took him in every time.

"He was cognizant up until three hours before he died. The Friday night before he died, my mother invited the whole family over to dinner. He wrote me a note personally and handed it to me there. How he wanted to be buried. He wanted to be buried in a traditional Jewish tachrichim, a plain white linen shroud, which swaddles the entire body, including the head and face. When a tachrichim is used, the coffin is kept closed.

"He wrote this all out for me on a piece of paper. He asked if I would take care of my sister, Ann, and my mother. He didn't ask it of anybody else. Just me. I remember receiving that note and trying not to cry at the dinner we were having, and I then went home and cried and cried.

"It still affects me," he says today.

The idea of holding meetings to share their headache treatment knowledge originated with Dr. Donald Dalessio, and Seymour followed up on it. The meetings were educational, as contrasted with theoretical or research oriented, and programmed to educate physicians and provide continuing education in headache diagnosis and treatment.

The first one was held in 1976 at the University of New Mexico. Several hundred physicians attended, and that first success influenced the American Association for the Study of Headache's board of trustees to continue holding the educational meetings. They held meetings in Tarpon Springs and San Diego at first, and then in 1979, they moved their annual educational meeting to a facility in Scottsdale, Arizona. In 1981, they began holding it at the Camelback Inn in Scottsdale. Seymour organized them all and taught at them as well.

"During my early years, I did hundreds and hundreds of lectures. Hospitals held clinical pathological conferences. Once a week they'd have a big conference at different hospitals and medical schools throughout the country. I was invited to speak—I did as many as ten to twelve talks per month. That's a lot. I really did a lot of traveling during those days!

"That's what built up my headache practice. I collected a lot of fountain pens and plaques," Seymour laughs. (Such gifts were typically presented to speakers.)

Not only did he teach in those speaking engagements, but he also learned a lesson or two along the way.

"In 1981, I was invited to lecture at the University of Illinois Medical Scholars Program. It was my lecture titled 'Stress and Feedback' with a biofeedback demonstration. When I arrived, I was happy to see that the lecture hall was full of students and their instructors.

"My standard set of slides featured a female—blonde, statuesque—wrapped only in a sheet. I advised the audience about the personality features of a typical migraine patient. She was between twenty and forty, very neat or organized, etc. I commented that it was because of the young lady featured in the slide that I enjoyed my work. Suddenly, about twenty female students (and some female instructors) walked out of the lecture hall.

"I continued with my lecture and eventually discussed the use of biofeedback in migraine therapy. At this point, I showed a slide of a cartoon. It depicted a woman, flat-chested but with a large derriere, reading a book about the power of positive thinking. In the next slide, she stands on her head, and when she becomes upright, she is now large-breasted with a small derriere. I noted that biofeedback could not perform miracles. Again, a group of women walked out of the lecture, accompanied by some of their male colleagues.

"At the end of my lecture, the professor who had invited me apologized for the disruption but begged me to understand the sensitivity of the audience. I later discovered that the female medical students had voted me 'Chauvinist of the Year.'

"I did learn from the experience and became more aware of gender sensitivity and political correctness in my lectures. My portfolio was edited for any offensive slides, and after that incident, I managed to keep my audience in their seats.

"A little aside: Presenting doctors today are supported in most instances by the pharmaceutical industry. They used to be sponsored by organizations or they'd present their information as an individual. There was no interest in the sponsorship that's prevalent today. People who spoke in those days did it for prestige and because they were in demand for educational purposes. Present day, not that they don't want them for prestige or educational purposes, but behind each speaker is usually pharmaceutical support, and there are many physicians who make their living doing this.

"To be a little more critical, there are many people going around lecturing on headache who do not have the same patient-oriented experiences—and I don't mean to be egotistical—which are so important in treating patients. They talk hypothetically about drugs without necessarily having the personal experience that somebody who actually treats patients and sees patients would have. Sometimes I get a very difficult case to work on, and I always try to emphasize that not everything works. It takes time. And one of my fortes is the use of various treatments together in combination that may help a patient. You have to get a certain feel for doing this."

During his ongoing campaign to build the membership base for the American Association for the Study of Headache, Seymour found that he wasn't able to keep up with the demands of this non-paying position and launch his own headache practice all by himself. The association agreed to hire a secretary to help him. After working with several others who ultimately moved on to other positions, Seymour's sister, Idell, wound up with the job of secretary.

"In fact, after I was beheaded, they kept her for several years afterward," Seymour recalls.

Beheaded?

"The Diamond Headache Clinic generated a lot of interest because nobody ever thought of having a private practice headache clinic. This was the first of its kind in the United States. In the past, they've been part of a hospital unit.

"It generated doctor interest, it generated public interest, and it generated a fair amount of ridicule from my colleagues. That happens whenever you do something different, and it took time to get rid of that attitude."

Medical specialization was not the norm in the early 1970s. Some doctors were narrowing their range of work, but as Seymour put it, "The general flow of thought in medicine was that the majority of doctors should be in family or general practice.

"There were residencies in surgery and medicine at that point," he explains, "but nobody ever thought to consider headache as a specialty. One of the prominent journals, *The New England Journal of Medicine*, in fact—after our headache clinic received some notoriety—wrote an editorial against 'overspecialization.' They felt that maybe this idea of specialization was being overdone, and they used my headache clinic as an example."

"When I opened the Diamond Headache Clinic, it generated interest among many doctors who thought that if my clinic was successful, they'd like to do the same thing. I was very gracious about sharing information; I didn't want to run a monopoly.

"Among my visitors was a group from Connecticut, a psychiatrist and a neurologist, and another group from Florida. They all wanted to spend time with me and see how the clinic functioned so they could set up similar operations. And I showed them everything.

"One of the people who came to see me was a young neurologist who was finishing his residency at the University of Michigan. He was very son-like to me and did everything in the world to ingratiate himself to me.

"He presented a couple of papers, which were of good quality, and he would call me every Sunday morning to talk with me about how he should handle certain things, both professional and personal.

"One of the personal things he told me was that his grandmother had died and left everything to the other grandchildren, leaving him out of the will. He asked my opinion of whether he should take it to court, to try to get his portion. After his phone call, I discussed it with Elaine, and she said I should be wary of him because no Jewish grandmother would disinherit her grandchild unless he was really bad.

"All of a sudden, I heard that some of my so-called friends were getting together to depose me from my position at the American Association for the Study of Headache. Among these were a lot of people I befriended, and leading them was the young neurologist!

"I knew something was going on. People who I thought would support me did not, and other people who were my supporters— which was a large group—were not vocal. They held a meeting near O'Hare International Airport in one of the meeting rooms at a hotel, and at the end of the meeting, it was concluded that I would step down after two years.

"I listened to the accusations; some of them were blatant lies. The whole thing felt like a conspiracy, you know. I was hurt, but I was also very gracious about it and said that would be fine. The disappointment and sadness over this betrayal bothered me for years.

"They assumed I was just going to back down and practice medicine and grow old and die. But I really didn't want to do that,"

Seymour smiles. "So I formed a new organization: The Diamond Research & Educational Foundation. We ran our first educational meeting through that organization in Cincinnati, Ohio. The meeting was run prior to the American Neurological Association and was highly successful. I invited my own speakers, and they came.

"It blossomed later into two successful annual meetings and eventually into three meetings every year. I ran a successful one-day meeting every year in Chicago. It usually coincided with the lighting of the Christmas trees along Michigan Avenue, which attracted young doctors and their families to attend. Then I ran the February meeting in Palm Springs. And finally, I ran a middle-of-July meeting at Disney World. Both the Palm Springs and Disney World meetings were three to five days in duration.

"You may wonder who would want to go to Florida in the middle of July. It's warm, it's humid, it's got bugs, and it rains every night. However, I accidentally stumbled onto the fact that many doctors with children suddenly realized that the summer was about to end, they hadn't spent time with their children, and they needed continuing medical education as well. So it served as a dual purpose. It was held at the Grand Floridian, a five-star hotel and the best on Disney's property. By the way, they're nice people to do business with, too!"

15. Growth and Expansion

Creation of the Diamond Headache Clinic had begun humbly in Seymour's family practice office, across from Rose Hill Cemetery, but it moved and expanded when Seymour became a real estate investor.

"When I was in family practice, I took care of a man who ran an electrical supply business not far from my office. His name was Leroy 'Roy' Jorgensen, and we became friends. He was also influential in referring me a great number of patients.

"Through Roy, I met Verne Oscarson, who was related to Roy's wife. One day after office hours, they invited me to have a drink. They imbibed heartily. I went out with them, and they talked about how they could build a nice medical building for me.

"Together, the three of us invested in the construction of a large building just south of my old office at 5212 N. Western Ave. Then, subsequent to that, I built another one. And then I built a third one where the clinic was eventually located, the ultimate headache clinic.

"The first and third were fairly large buildings, and the middle one was not very large because I didn't have the space, but altogether, the three buildings encompassed about two and a half blocks.

"I discovered that it's not good to be a landlord. I didn't manage the buildings—I had somebody else manage them—but I had a lot of tenants, and most of them were acquaintances or friends. So, if anything went wrong, they'd come to me. Eventually it became annoying enough that I sold them all."

Seymour continued working in his "ultimate headache clinic," renting it back from the individual to whom he sold it. Since he was the only medical doctor on staff originally, he devised ways to serve a larger number of patients with the help from his nursing staff. His nurses were trained to take a complicated medical history and to teach the patients about their medicine and management of their headaches.

"Nowadays, they have physician['s] assistants, but back then, nurses were nurses. I taught them to take a headache history. Taking a headache history is the most important thing you can do to make a diagnosis, and it's not as simple as just asking where their headache is. There's a proper sequence of questions they would follow. I had them printed on a card so they could run through it.

"We utilized these nurses to do headache histories, and they became very proficient at them. Anybody that worked for me for several years would become so proficient that they could come in and tell me—or I'd ask them to write down on paper what their opinion was—what type of headache the patient suffered, and so forth and so on. And they were better than 90 percent right because I had trained them that way.

"I remember that one of my nurses ... because of financial obligations, worked a part-time job at one of the hospitals as well. A patient came in to the hospital with a headache problem as well as some other issues.

"The resident in neurology at that time didn't know how to handle or diagnose the patient, but his nurse did. In my later communication with this doctor, he extolled how much this particular nurse knew.

"She told him what type of headache it was and how to treat it. My system worked so well and became so well known that other doctors came to visit our clinic to learn about it.

"The doctor visits continued up until about 2003. I stopped this due to the fact that it was being abused. Some doctors would say, even though they only spent two days at our clinic, that they were trained by me, and that's just not true."

Another project that publicized the Diamond Headache Clinic was Seymour's participation in Volume 33, Number 2 of the Ciba Symposia. The Swiss pharmaceutical company Ciba (now Novartis) published information provided by various medical sources for the benefit of all in a series of symposia.

In working on the paper, Seymour collaborated with well-known medical illustrator Frank Netter, whose *Atlas of Human Anatomy* is a medical treasure.

"I was honored to be asked to do it with Dr. Netter," Seymour recalls. "I went down to Florida to visit with him and go over what we needed. I believe he was around eighty years old at the time. He would play golf in the morning, and then he and I worked to integrate his drawings with my text in the afternoon."

Again in 1994, Seymour was invited to contribute an article to the symposia, and although Dr. Netter had died in 1991, Seymour again relied upon his illustrations to help convey his message.

As the Ciba Symposia transported Seymour's headache knowledge to physicians around the world, the credibility of Dr. Seymour Diamond and his Diamond Headache Clinic grew with each reading.

Within six months after opening his headache clinic, Seymour's appointments were set up months in advance, and in some cases patients had to wait for more than a year. To better manage the volume and get top-quality help to his patients sooner, he set up other new procedures.

Two individuals were assigned to manage appointments, one for new patients and the other for returning patients. Dr. Diamond also carried a card in his pocket that listed his available appointment times so that he could schedule revisits on the spot with his patients.

"Every day I insisted the receptionist make out a date list for my free times during the present month and months to follow," Seymour tells us. "It was a future appointment list, and I kept the list in a pocket of the lab coat I wore. And after I'd finished with a patient, I'd say, 'I want to see you in two weeks,' and take out the list and give them the specific day and time I wanted to see if they were available. This showed the patient my interest and concern about their outcome and established a relationship. Some of the people I taught to do this later neglected to follow this doctrine, and I really castigated them!"

Furthering the personalized service idea, he also arranged a call-in time each day when doctors would be available, and patients could phone the clinic and speak directly to their physicians (as the business grew, other qualified doctors were added to the staff).

Since they often worked with drugs that could be addictive if used improperly, he initiated a policy that required patients to obtain approval before receiving refills. When dealing with pain patients, open-ended prescriptions can easily cause addiction.

Along with that policy, he tried to manage other cases where patients didn't take their medications and didn't schedule appointments. For that problem, he set up a room with a telephone that became known among the nurses as "the torture chamber." Every day, a nurse was selected in rotation to review the patient charts and call the patients to assure that all medications were being taken according to doctor's orders. The torture chamber moniker reveals that it wasn't a favorite duty among the nurses, but with this system, patients could be assured that a knowledgeable person was always available to them.

Seymour also provided an on-site psychiatrist to help evaluate patients. The Minnesota Multiphasic Personality Inventory (MMPI) was administered to determine the individual's personality structure and psychopathology. In addition, they used a form provided by Princeton University to make a system evaluation of the GI and other bodily functions. All was taken into consideration when making a headache diagnosis.

"Among medical schools and large clinics, a thing called polypharmacy was an enigma," Seymour adds. "In other words, they were very critical of anybody who used multiple drugs. There's a fallacy in that … patients can have more than one kind of headache and more than one coexistent disease. So, more than one drug might be effective in preventing their symptoms, or they may have different degrees of pain, which might need a different level of analgesics. Different types of analgesics (pain relievers) for different symptoms.

"So I constructed a new word. Whenever I gave my lectures, I said, 'Instead of *poly*pharmacy, let's call it *co*pharmacy.' That was a more realistic approach and didn't have the years-long taint of the medical institution about using more than one drug. In other words, I wasn't going to go out on a campaign against the stigma of polypharmacy; I just created a new word.

As with Seymour's general practice, affiliation with a hospital to assist in severe cases, especially for out-of-town patients, became necessary for his headache work, too.

"I developed a very large headache practice and was about six months behind in seeing new patients unless they suffered from an imminent, organic disease or a cluster headache patient who needed immediate help.

"At the same time, I felt that there was a group of patients who[m] I could not satisfactorily treat. These were patients who had been improperly treated by other physicians and who were taking excessive over-the-counter and prescription headache medicines not meant to be used on a daily basis, and were developing what we call a rebound headache.

"In other words, they were taking these medicines, and then they would go off them. It wasn't an addiction to the medications; it was a rebound reaction from taking too much medicine. These patients were difficult to treat on an outpatient basis. There were other needs for hospitalization of headache patients, too: Chronic cluster headache patients who were unresponsive to therapy, patients who have a physician-induced habituation, and patients who could not be successfully treated without daily management. Another reason why this was important is that many of our patients came from out of town, and we needed a facility to monitor them.

"So, in 1981, in conjunction with the board of directors and the administration, I opened a small fourteen-bed unit at Bethany Methodist Hospital in Chicago. They agreed to give me a private area. It wasn't the best, by the way; it was a section they hadn't been using too much.

"I established the unit at that point. They gave me space away from the unit to do my biofeedback treatment and other therapies because I wanted that to be an integrated part of my program.

"I stayed at Bethany Hospital for three years. I kept the unit fairly busy, although not 100 percent busy, but they reneged on their pledge that they would keep the unit separate from other doctors' patients. When they would have a surge of flu or other serious respiratory illnesses where they needed the beds, they would admit other non-headache patients. But certainly in a closed unit like mine, I didn't want to have so-called healthy patients mixed with the people who had contagious disorders.

"There was also a lack of understanding about what I was doing, what I was trying to accomplish with the unit, and there grew a great deal of antagonism by some influential staff members against the unit.

"They didn't want my patients there. They thought I was a nut.

"Subsequently, around late 1982, I was approached by Mortimer Zimmerman, who was a well-known hospital administrator from Weiss Memorial Hospital. Weiss Memorial was a prestigious hospital, well-known for its surgical excellence. It was affiliated with the University of Chicago Medical School and Hospital.

"We met, and at that time, managed care had become a large factor in hospital admissions. In other words, the government (Medicare) and the insurance companies were doing everything they could to discourage hospital admissions.

"The government had committees to approve admissions, to determine whether they were valid, and the insurance companies usually followed Medicare recommendations because it saved them money. It wasn't right, but it was done that way.

"Weiss offered me a large unit on the fifth floor separated completely from the rest of the hospital. It was my area. There wouldn't be any interference in any admissions, no matter how busy they got. Mr. Zimmerman also said that he would build it to my specifications. The only drawback was that I only had one private room on the floor.

"It was a twenty-eight-bed unit, and they constructed a separate biofeedback unit for me within the unit. My daughter Judi, who is an architect, and I worked together to design a floor layout that would best serve my patients. The unit prospered, not only financially but in reputation during that time. They also provided some funds for us to use for educating doctors regarding headache.

"By the way, before I left, Bethany offered me a paying job on their board of trustees to get me to stay, but I was more interested in what I could accomplish than anything personal, and so I had no qualms in moving the unit. We moved to Weiss in 1983 and stayed there until 1993.

"One of the convenient things about Weiss is that they owned a large apartment building adjacent to the hospital where families from out of town would be able to stay at a nominal rate while their relative was being treated.

"We had a wonderful relationship, even with the managed care people, because I was allowed to sit down and discuss the necessity of each admission with the physician chairman. I didn't have the constant fight that I might have had in other places about the authenticity of each admission."

The term "managed care" refers to a highly controversial system created to reduce the cost of health care. According to a book entitled *The Social Transformation of American Medicine*, U.S. President Richard Nixon was an early advocate of a system that would change American health care from its not-for-profit business model to a for-profit plan that would be driven by the insurance industry. The Health Maintenance Organization Act passed in 1973 encouraged the growth of HMOs (Health Maintenance Organizations), an early form of managed health care.

In short, advocates claim that managed care has curbed health care costs while critics claim that it hasn't succeeded in that goal because health care expenses have surpassed the GDP (Gross Domestic Product) by almost 2.5 percent since 1970, and there are many claims that necessary care has been denied, even in life-and-death situations, or that low-quality care has been substituted for quality care, all in the interest of cutting costs.

Regardless of opinion—public as well as professional—about 90 percent of insured Americans are enrolled in some sort of managed care program today.

Seymour got his chance to voice his criticism of managed care before a large audience when one of the major TV networks felt that his headache clinic would provide a unique and interesting story for its viewers.

"One of the people they were filming was a patient I was taking off an abused drug given to her by a doctor. They interviewed her, and while they were doing it, she suffered a seizure. They filmed it, and I explained to them at the time that we probably did the withdrawal (this was a medicine, a prescribed medicine) a little too fast, but we were hampered in what we could do because managed care hadn't allowed enough time to do it safely."

By the early 1990s, Mortimer Zimmerman had left Weiss Memorial Hospital, and the University of Chicago had appointed a new administrator as well.

"The new administrator wasn't the most understanding or sympathetic person to what we were doing," Seymour recalls. "He had conferences about cutting whatever budgets we had for doing things. He wanted to cut our educational programs, both for the patients and what we did as far as education for physicians in headache treatment. Basically, we left because of the antagonism that developed with this new administration.

"And one other point: Weiss was one of the largest surgical hospitals with a gigantic, prestigious staff when we were there. But by the time I was ready to leave, it had dwindled in its prestige, its business, and its hospitalizations because the new administration failed to realize the importance of cardiac surgery. This was an exciting time in cardiology when they developed the bypass operation and other important advances. But abdominal surgeons controlled the hospital, and they didn't realize that a whole new avenue was opening up in medicine."

It was time to change hospitals again and, fortunately, opportunity once again arrived just in the nick of time.

"My daughter Merle had done part of her residency at Columbus Hospital," Seymour recounts, "and I received a call from one of the administrators saying they would like to have lunch with me.

"They wanted to build a unit for me to my specifications. They agreed to have my daughter Judi draw the plans in conjunction with me. And they wanted to supplement our educational budget, both for patients and also for general education about headache.

"I called my lawyer about this and we met. Marvin Cohn was a good friend, a cluster headache patient, and also volunteer counsel for the National Headache Foundation. He did a lot for us during this time, and he was a good friend of mine—one of my best friends. He was a good attorney, and he was sincere. We entered into a two-month negotiation with the hospital, and we got a very attractive package.

"I was a pretty bad driver. Not that I didn't know the rules or anything else, but at that time, my mind would wander on different business and medical things, and just prior to the negotiations, I'd almost had a very serious accident that could have killed me. It was that serious. And part of the negotiations that Marvin Cohn worked out was that they would provide a car for me. I would pay whenever they would provide a driver, but I would only pay for the time that he spent in driving me. Just on a personal note, it was nice to have the car, especially when I went to the medical school to lecture, a good two-hour drive. It had its inconveniences because I always had to wait for the driver, but it provided me with a lot of time to do my writing and do things for the hospital unit, the hospital, and the practice.

"So, we worked out the deal. It took about seven months to build the unit. I did not renew the contract with Weiss Memorial Hospital, and we moved to Columbus Hospital. They couldn't have been more gracious.

"Columbus was a Catholic hospital, and I had seen several of the sisters as patients in my clinic previously. So there was a nice relationship. The unit was excellent; it provided me with more resources to use.

"Our unit is special. There's nothing like it in the world. They provided me with the new contract, the incentive, the support, and the encouragement to build a unit like no other could ever be. Could *ever* be. Nobody trying to duplicate our effort could encompass the services we had. They helped me provide a once-in-a-lifetime type of hospital unit.

"We moved there in 1993, and one of the things that was very fascinating about this hospital was their shrine. Within the hospital, they had a shrine that was comparable to the wonderful churches you might see in Europe. It was big; I think it could hold about three to four hundred people."

Columbus Hospital was founded in 1905 by St. Frances Xavier Cabrini and the Missionary Sisters of the Sacred Heart of Jesus—Stella Marie Province. Also known as Mother Cabrini, she was the first U.S. citizen to be canonized by the Roman Catholic Church. She was born in Italy in 1850, one of eleven children born to Agostino Cabrini and Stella Oldini. Cabrini took her religious vows in 1877 and became Mother Superior at the House of Providence orphanage. After the orphanage closed, she wrote the rules and constitution of the newly formed Missionary Sisters of the Sacred Heart of Jesus. She earned the attention of Pope Leo XIII when the sisters established a free school, nursery, and seven homes.

Mother Cabrini wanted to establish new missions in China and went to the Vatican for approval, but instead, the Pope sent her to America to help the Italian immigrants who lived there. She and six other sisters arrived in New York in 1889, where they founded the orphanage Saint Cabrini Home in West Park. It would be the first of sixty-seven institutions she founded across the U.S. as well as South America and Europe.

While still in New York, she founded Columbus Hospital and Italian Hospital. In Chicago, the Sisters opened Columbus Extension Hospital, which was later renamed Saint Cabrini Hospital. Mother Cabrini died in 1917 at the age of sixty-seven of complications from dysentery. She was canonized in 1946 by Pope Pius XII. Her shrine was dedicated in 1955, thirty-eight years after her death.

"Whenever I had pharmaceutical visitors or doctors interested in our unit, I would take them, besides seeing our hospital unit, to see the shrine," Seymour reminisces.

"In the meantime, our unit prospered. It was a thirty-bed unit; we kept it completely filled and always had a waiting list for patients to come in.

"Around 1999, hospitals were having difficulty in filling beds because of managed care being very strict. The insurance people were making very restrictive rules about who should be hospitalized and how long they should be hospitalized.

"Economic difficulties occurred at these hospitals, and it was decided that St. Joseph's Hospital and Columbus Hospital would merge. St. Joe is a beautiful hospital on the lakefront. And again I went into negotiations with them.

"I formulated a contract that improved what we had. First of all, we would take an entire floor, about thirty-eight beds, which is a lot. And they were built as all-private rooms, each with its own bathroom, and a good majority of the rooms faced the lake.

"They built special lecture facilities and offices for my auxiliary personnel. They built everything that anyone could ever dream about having and provided a large educational budget as well.

"We built a biofeedback unit that could treat five patients at any one time, and part of our program was that patients would have biofeedback twice a day. The hospital helped provide training for the people who ran it for me.

"We even had an art instructor as part of the unit so that people could do art therapy and other things. We had a conference room with a large TV and films that I had done, a series of films about different headaches and their treatments.

"We had a dedicated dietician because—and some of my colleagues would argue—about 30 percent of headache sufferers are affected by what they eat. The dietician would give lectures to our patients about how foods affect their conditions.

"And contrary to what most hospitals had, I secured in my new contract a registered pharmacist dedicated to the unit. If the patient needed pain medication or other medicine, it could be administered immediately rather than hours later. We hired Richard Wenzel, Pharm.D., who has successfully developed a program teaching the patients about their drug therapy. He now has pharmacy students who travel from throughout the U.S. to learn about headache treatment. The presence of a pharmacologist on the unit has certainly improved patient outcomes.

"We also had our own physical therapy area, so we didn't have to send patients to a different floor. We have several areas for physical therapy. This is a big floor I took over!

"Then, on the same floor, we built a seven-room unit for relatives. It was very cleverly designed so people could not directly go from there to see the patients. They would go through the reception area, where they could be checked in appropriately.

"And finally, we had an exercise area with a bicycle and a treadmill to encourage patients to exercise.

"Our unit couldn't be duplicated today. Budget, or the amount of effort, or the confidence for something like this being viable ... it just couldn't happen today.

"I also negotiated that we would have some input over the nursing and auxiliary nursing staff on the floor. You know, this is something I'm really proud of. This is something nobody else has in the world. We also negotiated that we would have the right to train the personnel, that the personnel we selected would be dedicated to the unit. And let me qualify that: If administration started shifting nurses around, they wouldn't have the understanding of the type of patient that we supported. As a result, our nurses were cross-trained so that there was always a nurse who was knowledgeable about headache working on our floor.

"What I'm trying to say is that we need people working on the floor who understand headache and its treatment. We do not need people oversolicitous or sympathetic. This is some of my own research. I found when family members and caregivers become oversympathetic and keep asking about the pain or the headache or the trouble they're having, it may compound the problem. It becomes a mechanism, a way of attracting attention, of making them important. I once wrote a paper on what they call the 'concubine syndrome.' And in this paper, I described multiple cases where a husband, wife, or a parent will overly use the oversolicitation and sympathy to actually control the patient, to keep them dependent on them.

"Patients couldn't leave the hospital for any reason, although many of them were mobile. I didn't want to get an interpretation from managed care that we weren't dealing with serious problems. I did provide for a group walk once a day in Lincoln Park.

"We established a daily program of classes for patients. For example, our dietician would talk two or three times a week, the pharmacist would talk, we offered yoga and tai chi. The nurses would talk about their work with the patients. There would be a set program, at least three or four classes a day. And biofeedback training occurred twice daily.

"Once a week, we would have a session called 'Doctor's Bag,' when one of the physicians would be available to a whole group of patients in this large recreation area and answer any questions they had about treatment. The questions were not specific about themselves, but in general about headache, about pain, about anything they want to know. I used to love doing them myself.

"I want to mention that various people have seen the unit and then attempted to duplicate it. But there's nothing comparable to our unit as far as I know in the United States. There's nothing even close.

"In our early inpatient units, although smoking was banned throughout the hospital, we always included a dedicated 'smoking room.' A large contingent of acute and chronic cluster headache patient were smokers. If we hadn't provided them an opportunity to smoke, they would have refused inpatient treatment. The special area for smoking did not contaminate the rest of the hospital; however, with stricter state and city laws, the smoking rooms were eliminated.

"We've had a few bumps along the way. Our contract has come up a couple of times, and there's been major disagreement. My original contract went well because they wanted us very badly. Once we were there, as with many organizations, they then looked to save money. So, basically, we've had some renegotiations, some conflict, but it has worked out.

"One of the big worries ... any hospital has is dealing with managed care. I'm talking about Medicare; however, I want to qualify that. The number of Medicare patients we serve is only about 8 or 9 percent of our patients because headache is not a disorder of old age as much as in younger ages. And one of the things I originally negotiated—and I did this before at Columbus—is that we have our own managed care department.

"Part of my contract states that two registered nurses from the clinic would work with managed care. In present day society, if you want to admit a patient, you have to call the insurance company or the Medicare office and get permission.

"Basically, we would call, for example, Blue Cross Blue Shield of Illinois, and we'd explain the reasons our patient should be admitted for hospital care. Typically, we would talk to a nurse who works for the insurance company, and many times she would give you authority, but many times she would say, 'I will have to put it up for review by a physician.' Once we got approval, the patient would be admitted, and they were defined by managed care—whomever it may be—UnitedHealthcare, the government, Blue Cross Blue Shield, Anthem, or any of these companies. The patients were assigned to a certain number of days. They would usually give three to five days, which most times wasn't sufficient for our needs. It usually takes about seven or eight days to be effective. There are some people who have what we call status migraine, who[m] we can help in three or four days, but others aren't as fortunate.

"So I established what I call my own managed care, with hospital support because it's expensive, with two registered nurses having a special office on our floor. They would check on the status, reassure the patient, talk to the managed care people, and they had to be fluent in understanding why a patient was in the hospital and why we wanted to keep them. Over the years, these nurses have built up a relationship with the different managed care companies, which makes our work much easier. Most insurance companies considered the Diamond Headache Clinic inpatient unit a 'practice of excellence,' which made hospitalization and extended stays in the hospital easily approved.

"The next thing I want to mention is the offices on our floor. I had my personal office, a second office up there, which was beautiful. We also had offices for two psychologists, and two psychiatrists. And an office for our nurse who ran the floor, the supervising nurse, Barbara Gary, who has been with me since I opened the inpatient unit at Weiss. She was dedicated to our floor.

"We employed the psychologists and psychiatrists. In the difficult patients we see, there's always some psychological or psychiatric background. These are difficult patients. The majority of patients we see are not the average ones—the ones we hospitalize are not the average run-of-hospitalization patients, not typical headache patients. They could not be properly managed on an outpatient basis.

"Many of these patients would go on to lives of habituation, addiction, and chronic pain if we were not available to interfere and break it up. Managed care people and doctors who have a realization of this problem should be referring us work instead of monitoring us. With their computers, the insurance companies could certainly sort out the headache patients who are drug abusers. It would certainly be more economically feasible to refer these patients for appropriate treatment rather than to continue their addictions."

16. Mary Franklin

"She knows me almost as well as my wife does," Seymour has said more than once about his nurse extraordinaire of more than four decades, Mary Franklin.

When she began working at the family practice shared by Doctors Baltes and Diamond, Mary was a recent graduate, a registered nurse who had tried her hand at a Johns Hopkins nursing position in Baltimore but returned to her native Chicago after only two weeks, homesick and unhappy with her first job. And thus began her search for another job in Chicago, which would ultimately introduce her to Dr. Seymour Diamond.

"I answered a want ad in the paper. Dr. Diamond's partner, Dr. Baltes, interviewed me, so I didn't meet Dr. Diamond until my first day of work. I was twenty-one years old, and this was my second nursing job. I started September 20, 1970," she recalls.

And what was her first impression of Seymour?

"He was like a bull in a china shop. There must have been a hundred patients that came through that Monday. And this was the family practice. Headache patients accounted for a very small portion of our work then. Dr. Baltes wasn't in the office that day. I think he was on a trip somewhere, so Dr. Diamond was there by himself."

And what was his first impression of her?

"What the hell did you hire her for?" Seymour asked Dr. Baltes when he learned of their new employee. It wasn't that he questioned her capabilities; it's just that Dr. Baltes hadn't consulted with him before bringing in the new nurse, and he was surprised by the decision.

"I was hired to replace a nurse who was going on leave," Mary confides with us today.

She continues, "They let me start by writing prescriptions. Dr. Diamond would tell me what I was supposed to give the patient, and he would rattle medications off at a fast pace. I didn't know diet pills. You don't use them in the hospital, and I don't think we ever learned about them in school, except that they were bad.

"He had ordered something, and I started to write the prescription, but then he said something else, and I didn't recognize it as another diet pill. But the patient knew, so she went to the head nurse and mentioned it to him, and he started screaming at me. I said, 'You know, I'm used to taking care of sick people. I'm not used to taking care of fat people who come in for diet pills!'

"It was like that for about the first six months. My friend Veryl Gambino, who was my roommate at the time, used to give me pep talks on Wednesdays because on Wednesday they didn't see patients. Dr. Diamond would be there by himself in his office, and you were expected to run in every time he yelled. And just like today, if he doesn't have something to do, he's going to make your life miserable. So Veryl would say to me, 'You're going to be okay. You had nuns in school; this is no worse than the nuns. It's just like the nuns yelling at you.'

"One day, Dr. Diamond was standing in the reception area, taking a call from home. When he hung up, he turned to me and said, 'Merle got 610 on her SATs in English!'

"I made the mistake of saying, 'Oh, that's what I got, too.' And from then on, I was loaded with new types of work. He'd say, 'Come on ... you can do it, you can do it, you can do it!'

"You know, the years stretched out, and I didn't want to leave. I liked the people I worked with. It wasn't just working for an office. It was just a very vital place. There was research going on, the headache practice was growing. But I really loved the family practice. We had families where we took care of great-grandma and we took care of the new babies. So we saw the whole gamut. Sometimes it was sad, you know, when patients died or when they were diagnosed with something serious.

"But it was a really good job. It was always active, and I also realized that Dr. Diamond had a lot of respect—he would drive you crazy—but he had a respect for your opinion. And if I asked him something ... he didn't know, he would look it up. Despite the yelling, he treated everybody with respect concerning their opinions and patient care, and that meant a lot to me.

"And I just liked him! He started taking care of my family. He was my mom's main doctor until she passed away. He took care of my grandma. The patients were so loyal to him. They weren't that loyal to Dr. Baltes. If Dr. Diamond got mad at you, he got mad at you and then he forgot. Dr. Baltes held grudges. I can remember Dr. Baltes threw a chart at me one time and I almost walked out, but Dr. Diamond talked me into staying.

"If Dr. Diamond had done it, I'd have thought, 'All right, that's just his mood.' But he was ... in his own funny way, he was respectful of us. And he thought nurses were smart and they could do things. And that's why I stayed at first.

"Then he got into biofeedback, and I had the opportunity to go to the Menninger Clinic with him. That was the summer of 1972. When we returned, he let me run the department. I also started doing research and writing with him. I could finally use some of the creative work that the nuns had instilled in me, and it just got easy. It got easy to come to work and not leave."

Seymour adds, "Mary was essential in creating a world-class biofeedback setup. She originally went with me and helped me in my investigations of biofeedback, and then made our clinic the primary and largest biofeedback center in the world. We use it avidly both in our inpatient and outpatient cases.

"And she's edited many of my books. I've written about thirty-six books, and she has written three of my mass media books with me. She's very valuable, as far as I'm concerned," he concludes.

"I was sad when he stopped doing the family practice," Mary adds. "That was hard, but you know, I got used to the headache patients. And with a lot of them, we saw their families, too. You know, the moms would come in and then the daughters. I got attached to quite a few of them.

"Then, probably in 1975—I'd been there about four and a half years—the woman who had been Dr. Diamond's head nurse for years left the practice. She knew him when he was at Illinois Masonic, so she'd been there forever, and she left. There was another nurse who had worked there before I showed up. I was running biofeedback, and he didn't want to give me the whole thing because she would have been really upset. So we shared the responsibility of being head nurse. Then she got hurt in an accident and quit, and I became main head nurse. And I did that until I left for maternity leave.

"The day I was leaving for maternity leave—I'll never forget this—my ex-husband drove me to the clinic, and Dr. Diamond's youngest daughter Amy was standing outside, sobbing. She had been working as the receptionist for the summer. The regular receptionist was on maternity leave.

"I got out of the car, and Amy was saying, 'I'm never going in there. I'm never speaking to him again. I hate him … blah-blah-blah … '

"I said 'Amy, we've got two hundred patients coming in!'

"'I don't care,' said Amy.

"So I said, 'Well, just come in the building.' And she decided to stay. I'll never forget that. That was my last day before going on maternity leave. Oh, my God, that was a nightmare. She was quitting, and she was never going to speak to him again!

"Oh, he's mellowed now. And I don't even know what he'd said to set Amy off, but they'd had a real fight and she was quitting.

"Then I went on maternity leave, and I started typing reports for him at home. He eventually got me back in the office, and I was working three or four days a week. I would be home with the baby, and I'd get a call, 'So-and-so called, and you have to come in.'"

Seymour remembers her son Tim, who is now a successful lawyer, with a grandfather-like pride. "When he was four years old, they enrolled him in a Jewish preschool. And they went around to all the kids and asked them what was special about their mother. Timmy's answer was, 'She works for Dr. Diamond.'"

Mary resumes, "And then his longtime secretary quit. He had a couple secretaries, and he became aggravated with them. So he called me one day and said, 'What if you come in and help me with the administrative part?' I was just working as a staff nurse at that time. And I said, 'OK, but I'm only going to work three or four days a week.' 'Ok, fine,' he said.

"Well, within four months, I was working full-time, and that's when I went into the administrative part. That was in 1979."

Ironically, it was never Mary's intention to become a nurse.

"It wasn't anything I ever really wanted to do. My mother talked me into it. No, I'm a frustrated history teacher. Dr. Diamond encouraged me to go back to school. I do have my history degree. I got that in 1995 from Northwestern University. But I would have had to leave the clinic, so I never went on to get my teaching certificate or do student teaching. Then I got my master's degree in Chicago Studies. I did all my elective work in [the] history of immigration. He encouraged me to go back to school to do something.

"I actually only worked as a nurse at the clinic for about nine years, and then I got into administration. First, I was administrative assistant, then I was an administrator, and finally I wound up being VP of administration and publishing.

"About that time, anything that was being published by the clinic landed on my desk for proofreading, editing, and writing, too. Then he and I wrote a book. The first book was a consumer book on headache called *Coping with Your Headaches*. Then, he started *Headache Quarterly* in 1990, and I wound up being managing editor. I learned a lot from Amy (Seymour's journalist daughter) about editing.

"Did he tell you the biofeedback story?" she wonders. "This was one of his first encounters with Barbara Walters. She wasn't on the *Today Show* or anything like that at the time. It was when biofeedback was getting a lot of publicity, and they invited him to go to New York.

"I showed him how to put the biofeedback equipment on someone because he didn't do it himself, of course, we did it. So I showed him how, and I was sitting at home with Veryl watching. I got everybody watching the TV show, you know, Dr. Diamond's coming on! It was something similar to the *Nightline* show, but that wasn't it. It was a late-night show.

"And when Dr. Diamond put the biofeedback headband on Barbara Walters, he got it so tight I thought her eyes were going to pop out! I was screaming at the TV, and I could see she was going to say something like, 'This is supposed to help people?'

"When he returned to the office, he asked me, 'How did I do?'"

"I said, 'You almost killed her! What were you thinking?!'"

"But he'd do a lot of local TV. He was always getting calls to do local television, and he was always going places to lecture. He was terrible at driving. One time, I did rounds with him at St. Joseph's, and we were going back to the clinic. He was in that little Mercedes, and as we were getting onto Lake Shore Drive at Belmont, he stopped to yell at me about something. And I'm like, 'We're going to get killed! Could you just drive and yell at me later?'"

"I said from now on (I wouldn't drive the Mercedes, but I said from now on), 'I'm driving your car or my car, but if I'm getting in a car, you're not driving. Sorry.'"

"This happened back when he was still with the American Association for the Study of Headache. He was so dynamic with them with the meetings and always looking for newer lectures. He kept this all going constantly."

Mary recalls Seymour's so-called "beheading" when he was ousted from the organization.

"I was very hurt for him. It was really painful. People that he trusted, that he considered friends, showed their true colors. They weren't his friends. Some I was surprised at; some I wasn't. They were very narcissistic. It was a painful time for him. It's like, you raise this baby, and then it goes away from you. There was drama involved with it, but to push him out like that was disgusting. It was hard on him.

"The hardest thing he ever faced, though, was the Rita Richter lawsuit [described in chapter 21]. That aged him so much. That was very, very painful. Merle was still working in the emergency room then, and I used to pray that this lawyer that Rita Richter had … I didn't want him to die, but I wanted him to get a kidney stone and have Merle be the person on call when he entered the ER for treatment. I really did."

Seymour adds, "Mary worked for me until I retired about four years ago. She stayed with the Diamond Headache Clinic for an additional three years, working for the doctors who took over the practice. I don't think they fully appreciated her management personality and other factors that made her essential to my practice, and to our personal relationship, over the years.

"She became a friend, a friend to me and my family. And maybe, I think, there was a move to separate me and my influence (through Mary) from anything to do with the clinic.

"As a result, I suggested she apply for a job opening at the National Headache Foundation. There were three other applicants who also were interviewed by foundation personnel, but Mary proved to be the best qualified among them."

"The opportunity arose at the foundation, and I took it," Mary continues. "The clinic had taken a different direction, and I wasn't needed in the same capacity as I had been with Dr. Diamond. They were very nice to me when I left." She now renders her services to the National Headache Foundation as director of operations.

One of Seymour's pet peeves is medical workers who refer to their medical doctor bosses using their first names. "It takes away from the dignified position of being a physician," he says. And on that score, along with many others, Mary Franklin once again sets the standard.

"In all the years we worked together—forty-two now, in 2012— she never called me Seymour. She called me Dr. Diamond or boss. And I appreciated it."

17. National Headache Foundation

S eymour was still working with the American Association for the Study of Headache when he recognized the need for an organization created primarily for lay people rather than physicians to promote headache education and sponsor research for new headache treatments.

"There was no organization like it in the U.S.," he states. "There was a British Migraine Society, so I went over to see what they were doing. By the way, they pronounce 'MY-grain' differently than we do; they call it 'MEE-grain.'"

Elaine and their three daughters accompanied him on the trip, and they stayed at London's renowned Savoy Hotel. Seymour spent a day with the man who ran the society, learning about his organization, and that evening Seymour invited him and his family to dinner. All was going smoothly at dinner, but then as they were discussing a successful mutual acquaintance that had moved to the United States from Great Britain, the man leaned close to Seymour and commented in a conspiratorial tone of voice, "He's a Jew, you know ... "

Elaine and the girls were taken aback but said nothing, and Seymour found a way to acknowledge the comment gracefully while moving on with the purpose of his visit. Despite yet another encounter with anti-Semitism, albeit a minor one, he gathered sufficient information to return to the U.S., where he began the fight to form his own organization.

It was an uphill battle because other AASH members opposed it, including the organization's treasurer, Robert Ryan. "Dr. Ryan in his usually fiduciary, peculiar ways, really strongly opposed it, but I had enough political say-so to get it done," Seymour explains.

Seymour eventually overcame their opposition, acquired seed money for the fledgling group, originally called the National Migraine Foundation, and established a small office where Elaine served as the sole (unpaid) employee. It was an inauspicious beginning for what would become a strong force in headache treatment support years later under its current name, the National Headache Foundation, but then the brand-new organization needed help getting off the ground.

"I was being a pioneer here, promoting responsive research and headache education. I was on a mission," Seymour explains. "But it was really a young organization, and we needed help to get it started. To publicize the group, we started a newsletter. It was not a newsletter about fundraising; it spoke about different topics in headaches. We gave the readers information about diagnosing different kinds of headaches. We gave them insight into new treatments or old treatments that might have gone out of popularity, or about what was wrong with some treatments that were available.

"And it was very well done! My friend Donald Dalessio not only edited the journal for the American Association for the Study of Headache, but he and his wife, Jane, helped our first editor, Ann Henry, put together this newsletter, too.

"I did the first editorial, and as the first president of the organization, I told the story of how it got started. One of the things I did there was initiate a program where the National Migraine Foundation would sponsor medical students, interns, and residents who have shown interest in headache problems to the American Association for the Study of Headache meetings so as to interest them in it.

"In that first edition, we also discussed Dr. G. S. Barolin of Austria, who got the most recent Harold G. Wolff award and who presented a paper on electroencephalograph, that's EEG. He reported that migraineurs had a particular pattern of EEG changes. Subsequent studies years later did not show this to be true."

There were some funny stories that came along with the formation of the new organization, too. Early on, when Seymour and Elaine comprised the entire staff, they found themselves becoming overwhelmed with its steady growth. They hired a young woman to assist.

"Around 1980, I was invited to Italy, to Florence. And the assistant we'd hired was a very religious Catholic woman, so she asked Elaine if we could bring back a small copy of the Pietà for her," Seymour recounts.

The Diamonds are Jewish, of course, so they asked her to describe the Pietà for them.

"It's Mother Mary holding the baby Jesus," she said.

"So, I—stupid Seymour—went to Florence," Seymour continues. "They have tons of curio shops, and I kept looking for the mother Mary holding a baby, but I couldn't find one!

"So finally I came across an English-speaking vendor, and I said to him, 'Do you have the Pietà with mother Mary and the baby?'"

As most Christians know, the Pietà is a Michelangelo statue, not of Mary with the living baby Jesus on her lap, but with the body of the adult Jesus after he'd been taken down from the cross cradled gently in her arms.

"The vendor looked at me strangely, and then replied, deadpan, 'I'll have Michelangelo make one for you,'" Seymour concludes with a chuckle. He then learned of the mistake and picked up a proper Pietà for his faithful but misinformed assistant.

Some of the financial assistance in forming the foundation came from donors who had benefited from Seymour's help.

One of Seymour's patients was a man named Fred Smith, whose father had founded a large chain of supermarkets. Smith came to the Diamond Headache Clinic after failing to find help for his headache problem with other doctors. Seymour hospitalized him for cluster headache treatment and applied a histamine treatment originated by Bayard Horton and further developed at the Diamond Headache Clinic.

Smith's father sat at his son's bedside every day during his hospitalization, and both were very grateful for the success of the treatment.

Aware of the need for support, Seymour invited the father to become a board member of the organization. He declined, and instead his son joined and provided enough seed money that they could then hire a full-time director for the organization.

They hired Suzanne Simons as director of administration and development, and she would lead the NHF through two decades of steady growth and accomplishment.

In 1987, the National Migraine Foundation was renamed the National Headache Foundation, and in May of that year, the organization held its first fund-raising event at the Terra Museum of American Art in Chicago. It was a low-key affair compared to the organization's more recent events, but it became the first of the annual events that contributed to the National Headache Foundation's success.

"Daniel J. Terra is the founder of Terra Industries," Seymour explains, "and he was a renowned collector of American art; Bellows and Marsh and all the people who did American art in the, I would say, the '20s to '50s. He had a small museum in Evanston, and then he moved it down to this magnificent space on Michigan Avenue. We arranged to do our first fund-raising benefit there."

By now, the organization had built momentum and was well on track to meet Seymour's expectations. They planned their second fund-raiser almost immediately to be held in the summer of 1987, this time catering more to the pharmaceutical industry by holding it in New York City.

"We raised about $31,000 at that one," he says. "We had a silent auction, cocktail hour, and then an elegant dinner. We had guests coming from all over, and we offered some pretty spectacular live auction items that were donated by supporters. We had a car that was donated by Fred Smith, we had a private sixty-one-foot yacht donated for a month with the crew, somebody donated half-ownership in a race horse, we had vacation cruises, and the list goes on.

"In that same year, I did an hour-long documentary for the Public Broadcasting System (PBS), titled 'Man's Ancient Enemy.' This is also the time we started to donate money for research projects. Before, we were an educational-type group. We donated $23,000 to three research projects between '87 and '88. We gradually increased that sum so that we eventually supported ten or fifteen projects every year. Many of them later developed into major projects sponsored by the National Institute of Health."

The National Headache Foundation continued to present its annual fund-raisers, awarding various deserving individuals an ongoing series of awards, such as the Layman Support Award, the Media Support Award, and the Professional Support Award. The professional award has gone to many of Seymour's peers, pioneers themselves in headache medicine. The media award has gone to a number of familiar names and faces we see regularly on our TV sets: actress Lee Grant received it in 1995, and others since include Larry King, Matt Lauer, and Ann Curry. Dr. Art Ulene, a TV personality as well as a physician, received the professional award in 1996.

As when he launched his private practice and went on a mission to form a base of patients, Seymour approached the formation of the NHF with the same determined whatever-it-takes attitude.

Thus, when an announcer from the Moody Bible Institute radio station became a patient and asked him to speak on the air about headache issues, Seymour joined the media.

He recounts the experience: "The only instructions that they gave me during my performance is that I could not use profanity or God's name in any way. In other words, I couldn't say, 'Oh, my God,' or anything like that. I did all right with that, but I had to concentrate to not be as glib as I normally was."

The program was called *Open Line*, and each show featured a guest speaker who then responded to listener phone calls. Seymour had been hindered by religious prejudice at various points in his life, but his Moody Bible Institute experience certainly was not one of them. The Jewish physician fit in comfortably among a group of guest speakers whose topics were almost exclusively based on the Christian religion, and Seymour's appearances to discuss headache help were very popular.

"By the way, I feel—and I've done hundreds, maybe a thousand radio broadcasts in my life, and I've done hundreds of television appearances—for me, the radio is a much easier medium to handle, less stressful for me, personally.

"As a result of my Moody radio broadcasts, I started to get patients from all over the United States and some from the

Philippines. It was like being on a major network to very ardent listeners. The thing that was great about them was that these were a group of people who were educated and amenable to receiving help.

"One of the people who contacted me after one of the Friday nights I appeared on this radio broadcast was Earl Sorensen. He was an executive vice president and chief operating officer at the H. D. Hudson Manufacturing Company. He called me about his wife, Phyllis.

"She came in to see me at the Diamond Headache Clinic, and she had what we would call today 'chronic migraine.' That is, she was getting severe migraines maybe ten or fifteen times a month, and also a daily constant headache.

"She was on a very popular drug at that time for pain relief known as Fiorinal. There were so few drugs available during that time, Fiorinal had become very popular, but it contained a barbiturate. One could become addicted, and she was. She was taking six to twelve of them a day … I think *one* a day is too many!

"I spent a long time talking to her and her husband, and convinced them that no treatment was going to work until she got off the daily habituating drug. So we slowly weaned her off the Fiorinal and replaced it with a mixture that I had named the Diamond Pain Reliever Medicine. It contained analgesic drugs but nothing habituating whatsoever. I made this mixture because it gave a certain illusion that it was going to help the pain because pain can be psychological as well.

"Then I gave her a trial on the tricyclic drugs—amitriptyline, drugs of that nature. But nothing was successful.

"Next, I decided, because of the recidivist nature of her disorder, to try her on an MAO inhibiter, a drug called Nardil. She was somewhat helped, but not to the extent that either she or I were satisfied.

"At that time in my research in using the MAOs, I encountered a Dr. Shuckitt, a psychiatrist at the University of California. He had written about the use of tricyclic drugs with the MAO inhibiters used in combination for selective psychiatric diseases.

"If you read the package label of either drug, there are warnings saying that you can't do that, but he reported on a large series of his own patients who were difficult, where he had used a tricyclic/MAO inhibitor combination without getting the side effects. And the side effects can be massive. They can have a malignant hypertension stroke and sudden death. He felt the warning was overexaggerated. And [at] that time, I had tried it selectively on a few patients with a great deal of success, but the patients had to be educated on its proper use.

"So I decided to use it on Phyllis Sorensen, and the results were miraculous!

"As an aside, the Diamond Headache Clinic still uses these combinations. We have used it on hundreds of patients, being very selective on whom we use it on, giving people proper instructions, and we've never run into a problem. There is a large subset of patients who could be helped by the combination of drugs—a regimen that I initiated at the Diamond Headache Clinic.

"Phyllis became a regular patient of mine. They traveled in from Michigan. One day her husband asked if he could do anything for me, and I asked him if he would join our board of trustees. He joined and soon became the finance chairman. The Sorensens became good personal friends, and they were a great help in the formative years of the National Migraine Foundation, which later became the National Headache Foundation.

"I want to add something here. Among the most frequently used antidepressants today are SSRIs, selective serotonin reuptake inhibitors. But these are the Prozac-like drugs, and although many doctors may prescribe them for migraine and other headaches, they are virtually useless as compared to the tricyclic and MAO inhibitors."

About two years after he treated Fred Smith, his father called Seymour and invited him out to dinner. Seymour noted that the elder Mr. Smith exhibited slurred speech that evening (and he knew he didn't drink), so he called Fred and told him to take his father to a doctor. Sadly, the physician found an inoperable tumor, and shortly thereafter Fred's father passed away. In his will, he left one of the first endowments that the National Headache Foundation ever received, nearly half a million dollars in gratitude for the work Seymour had done to help his son.

That generous donation was topped by another patient, who Seymour describes in his book *Hope for Your Headache*

Problem—More Than Two Aspirin with a chapter titled "The Ex-Infantryman." The patient was called that because of his service in WWII. After Seymour provided a complex solution to his headache problems, they stayed in touch.

"We corresponded after he was better, and whenever he heard anything or saw anything about me, he wrote me a note and said, 'I hope you've seen this, Dr. Diamond. I'm always very appreciative of you, and I'm going to leave the National Headache Foundation a large contribution when I die.'

"Every year or two, I'd hear from him, saying that he's going to remember the National Headache Foundation. Then one day, I was in the foundation office talking to the administrator, and I said, 'You know, I think maybe we'll get a few hundred dollars from this man, but it's way in the future. I hope nothing happens to him; he's a nice man.'

"Then I received a call from a staff member who'd received a call from his estate representative saying that he left the foundation $2.2 million!"

One day, Seymour received a letter inquiring about the National Headache Foundation, the Diamond Headache Clinic, and what they were doing in research and education from a lawyer named Ronald Barnard. He identified himself as chairman of the Walter S. and Lucienne Driskill Foundation.

From the Driskill foundation's website: "Walter S. Driskill, along with his wife, Lucienne, ran a successful importing business for many years. The company, Dribeck Importers, Inc., headquartered in Greenwich, Connecticut, represented and imported Beck's Beer from Germany. Under the leadership of the Driskills, the business prospered. After the Driskills retired and moved from Connecticut to their home in Florida, their interest in philanthropy grew. In particular, the field of medical research and treatment attracted their attention. Also, they donated a building in Greenwich, Connecticut, to an organization known as Kids in Crisis" and continued to provide funds for it and several charitable organizations in the medical field, including two projects at Bethesda Hospital-Driskill Center for Caring Excellence and the Driskill Endovascular Center. "The Driskill Foundation is dedicated to furthering the goals and interests of Mr. and Mrs. Driskill."

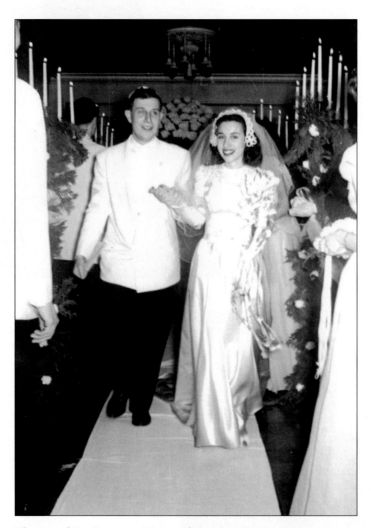

Elaine and Dr. Seymour Diamond, June 20, 1948

Mrs. Rose Diamond,
Dr. Seymour Diamond,
Mr. Nathan Diamond,
June 20, 1948

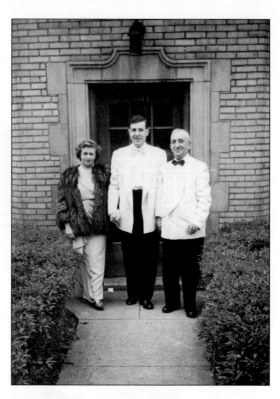

Dr. Leonard Lovshin and
Dr. Seymour Diamond,
late 1960s

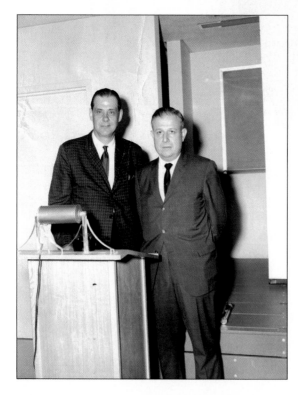

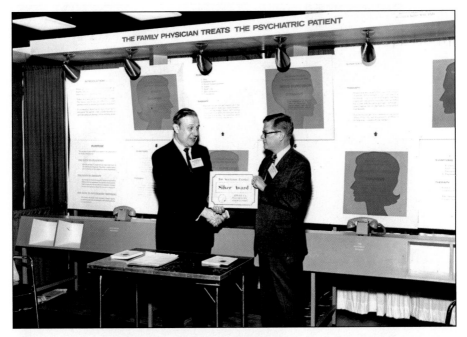

Dr. Seymour Diamond receiving Silver Award from the American Psychiatric Association, May, 1968

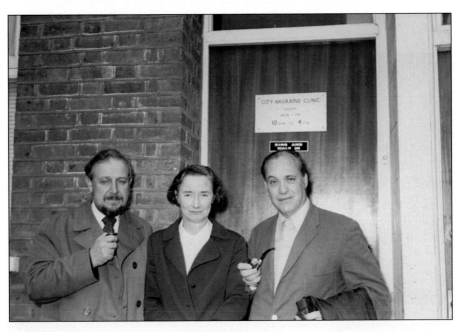

Dr. Seymour Diamond, Marcia Wilkinson, Robert Ryan Sr. at City Migraine Clinic, London, 1971

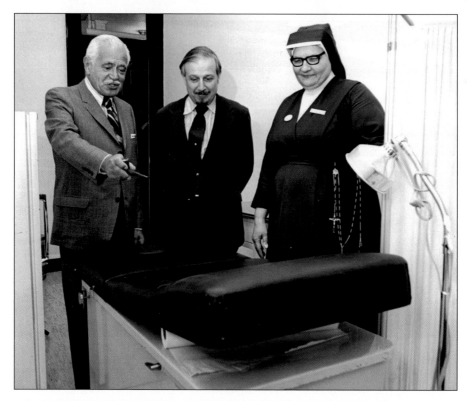

Dr. Irving Steck, Dr. Seymour Diamond, and Sister of Charity at the opening of DePaul Family Clinic in April, 1972

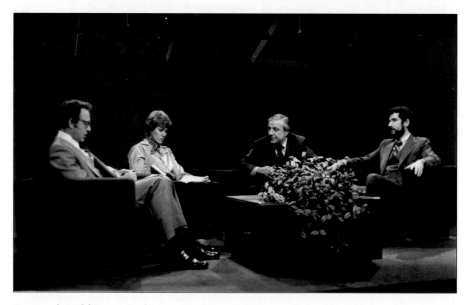

Dr. Frank Field, Lynn Redgrave, Dr. Seymour Diamond, Joe Graedon on the television show *Not for Women Only*, 1978

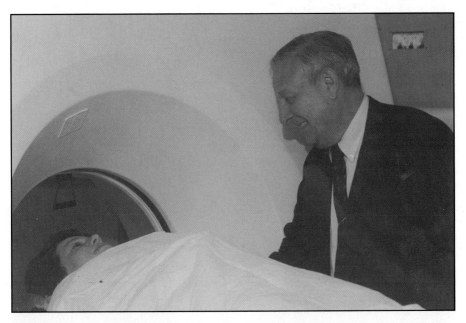

Dr. Seymour Diamond reassuring a patient undergoing a CT scan, 1986

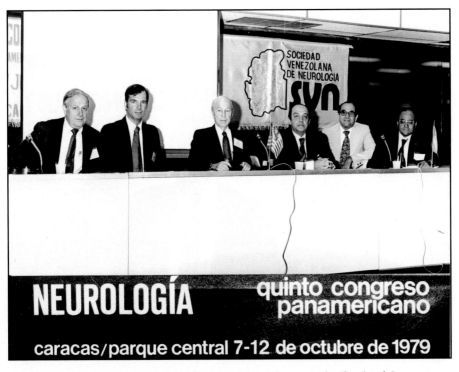

Dr. Seymour Diamond, Robert Kunkel Arnold Friedman, and officials of the
Pan American Neurology Conference

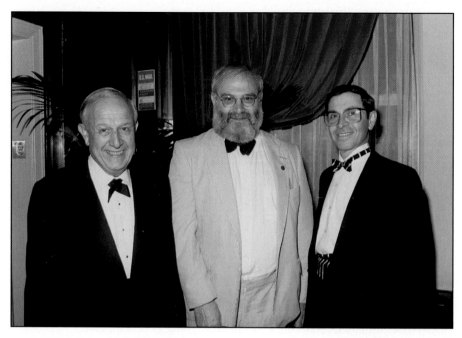

Dr. Seymour Diamond, Oliver Sacks, Arthur Elkind, 1991

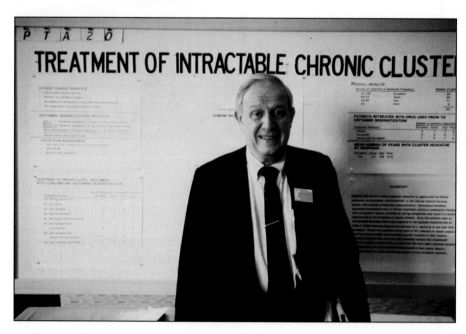

Dr. Seymour Diamond with poster presentation, 1985

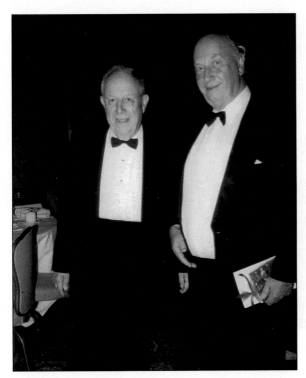

Dr. Seymour Diamond and
Sir John Vane, 1998

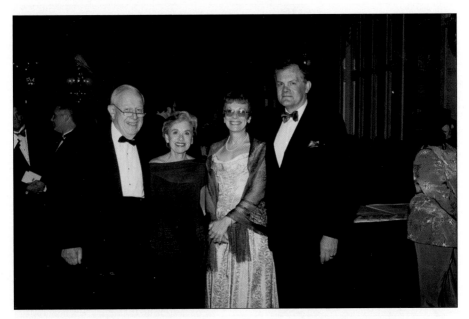

Elaine and Dr. Seymour Diamond, Mary and Dr. Patrick Humphreys, 1999

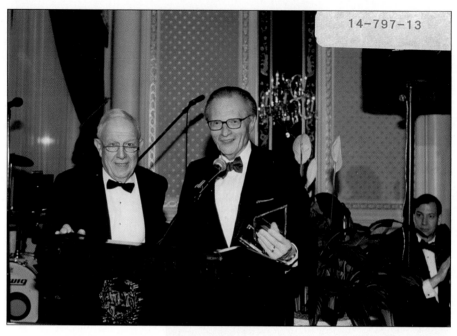

Dr. Seymour Diamond and Larry King, 2000

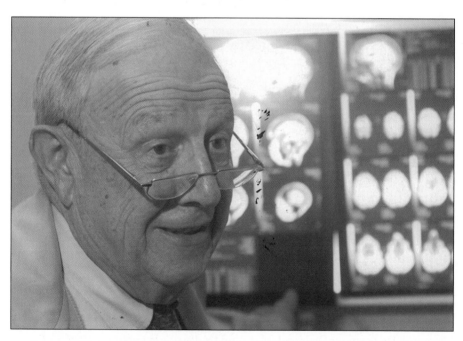

Dr. Seymour Diamond viewing MRI, 2000

Barnard asked Seymour to send him grant requests from the foundation as well as the clinic. Seymour and NHF legal counsel Jim Staulcup took a look at the foundation and saw that they had considerable funds available.

"But I didn't know what to request; I needed a ballpark figure," Seymour recalls, "so I called Ron and asked him. He said, 'That's up to you.' So then I asked him why he contacted me, but he responded, 'I'm not at liberty to tell you.'

"Anyway, I put in requests for more than I thought we'd get. I thought they could always give us less. I hadn't met him at that point, but we had fairly frequent phone conversations. We had a substantial request for the Diamond Fellowship and Educational Foundation. That's the one that supports the fellows at Loyola and at the clinic. It's a recognized fellowship, so after recipients finish their residency, they can take this fellowship, no matter what their specialty."

Seymour received a "substantial" amount of money for the Diamond Fellowship and Educational Foundation and a research grant for the National Headache Foundation as well. He and Barnard continued to communicate regularly, and a friendship soon developed.

"In fact, his wife volunteered to run our next benefit!" Seymour exclaims. "She and her daughter are in charge." He refers to the annual National Headache Foundation fundraiser, which in 2012 was held in Chicago at the Adler Planetarium.

But still, Seymour wondered of his good fortune with Mr. Barnard and the Driskill Foundation, why me?

"At one of our lunches, I asked him again why they picked me, and he told me a story," Seymour begins. "Mr. Barnard has a step-daughter, Katie Biggs. She went to the Diamond Headache Clinic for treatment, but her insurance was an HMO, and they wouldn't approve the course of treatment we'd designated for her.

"A physician from our clinic was kind enough to communicate with her family physician and guide him through a headache management program. That was Dr. George Nissan. He's no longer with the clinic. He's now at Baylor with another Diamond Headache Clinic alumnus, Dr. Freitag."

It was a stepfather's gratitude to a kind doctor for applying the Diamond Headache Clinic's attitude of caring for their patients' welfare that earned the two foundations the generous donations they received from the Driskills' foundation.

The National Headache Foundation got help from a number of concerned people during its formative years. Harold Levine provided financial assistance as well as his skills with producing the newsletter. Legal counsel was provided *pro bono* over the years by Leonard Rutstein, Marvin Cohn, and Jim Staulcup.

Harold Levine was originally research VP of Cooper Laboratories. He invented a headache relief medicine known as Midrin. Before the days of the triptans, his drug was of vital help for nonaddicting pain relief in headache patients.

Today's National Headache Foundation is a far cry from its early days. The website (www.headaches.org) offers educational opportunities for physicians and headache sufferers alike.

The organization's mission statement reads as follows: "To cure headache, and end its pain and suffering." Their vision is to have a world without headache. They aim to inform: "To serve as an information resource to headache suffers, their families, and the healthcare providers who treat them." To educate: "To raise public awareness that headaches are a legitimate biological disease and sufferers should receive understanding and continuity of care." And to "promote research into potential headache causes and treatments."

Also provided is a Physician Finder, where headache sufferers can find a doctor who is known to treat headache (it's noted on each entry whether the physician is "certified" or not).

The term "certified" refers to doctors who have earned a certificate of added qualification. While many patients are adequately treated by primary care physicians, some do require or seek more advanced care. For this reason, the National Board of Certification in Headache Management (NBCHM) was created to enable headache sufferers to identify these special physicians. The certifying process involves a peer-reviewed appraisal of qualifications reflective of a commitment to headache management. These qualifications and criteria include but are not limited to continuing medical education coursework in headache experience, headache patient caseload, and research.

The Our Community section of the NHF website connects viewers with a wide selection of human feedback and sharing, including a Facebook page, organized support groups, NHF blogs, and several other opportunities for headache sufferers to find help and share their burden with similarly minded others.

All has not gone exactly as planned, however, with the foundation, despite their best efforts. The National Headache Foundation replaced its executive director, Suzanne Simons, with a candidate whose primary directive would be to acquire funding for the foundation's various projects.

"I was in California last year when the foundation was moved to a new office space. When I came back, I was discussing my office with the architect, and I learned of some expenses that immediately set me off to look at the foundation's finances."

Seymour's review of the foundation's books appeared to show that more time had been spent enjoying executive perks than raising funds. As a result, the foundation first provided an opportunity to correct the situation, but when that failed, Seymour once again took the reins of the organization himself with Mary Franklin's assistance.

The National Headache Foundation continues its quest to increase public awareness and education for headache sufferers and their families. In addition to constantly improving its website, the NHF posts daily on Facebook and Twitter. In 2012, online chat rooms were introduced and are moderated by a thought leader in headache medicine. A variety of topics have been presented, including chronic daily headaches, pediatric headaches, post-concussion headaches and others. Each chat room involves fifty to one hundred participants, and the proceedings of each chat room is uploaded to the NHF website (www.headaches.org) as a podcast.

In 2011, the NHF launched a new quarterly magazine, *Head Wise*. Seymour, with the editorial committee of the foundaint, spearheads its publication. It has been welcomed by its readership as an excellent source for information on headache. Multiple copies are sent to physician members' offices to benefit even more patients and continue to raise awareness.

The NHF also continues to sponsor research into headache diagnoses and treatment. The foundation's research committee reviews applications from headache researchers throughout the United States.

18. Colleagues
Along the Way

Throughout his career, Seymour interacted with other physicians as well as those in the related fields and industry. These experiences influenced his life in various ways, both positively and negatively. As the clinic grew, new physicians were added to the staff—some successfully, some not.

Bernard Baltes

Dr. Baltes was a Ph.D./M.D.-educated pharmacologist whom Seymour met while working with the Riker Corporation, where Dr. Baltes was director of research. He was mentioned in earlier chapters. Dr. Baltes and Seymour parted ways when Seymour specialized in headache.

"Although Dr. Baltes was a tremendous help to me in establishing the validity and usefulness of the tricyclic antidepressants, I had already chartered the path. In 1963, I published an article in the *Illinois Medical Journal,* 'Use of Amitriptyline Hydrochloride in General Practice.'

"This led to my seminal article, 'Depressive Headaches,' which appeared in the journal *Headache* in 1964. Although it was the first mention of this form of headaches, this article is rarely cited.

"In 1966, in the journal *Psychosomatics,* I published the first article on the combination of a tricyclic antidepressant with a phenothiazine in the treatment of depression ('Double-Blind Controlled Study of Amitriptyline-Perphenazine Combination in Medical Office Patients with Depression and Anxiety'). This therapy is still utilized at the clinic for treatment of chronic daily headaches.

"With Dr. Baltes at the clinic, we were able to accept multiple invitations to lecture as well as contribute articles to the professional literature on our experience with the tricyclic antidepressants and their use in combination with other drugs. Because of my prior experience in nuclear medicine and Bernie's pharmacology background, we were able to tag amitriptyline with carbon 14, which enabled us to further explain the drug's actions.

"Dr. Baltes and I did an extensive study comparing the incidence of headache in a 'ghetto' clinic population, based on our experience at Mount Sinai Hospital on the west side of Chicago. We found that headache's occurrence was the same across all races and economic strata.

"Bernie and I remained in practice until 1974, when we split up and I focused my practice into strictly headache work. Bernie continued a family practice in Lincolnwood, Illinois. He and his wife, Marge, later moved to Arkansas, where Bernie maintained a small family practice and had more opportunities to fish and travel. He took care of Marge throughout her extended battle with lung cancer. Once he fully retired, he spent more time with his six children and many grandchildren. He was living with his oldest daughter when he was stricken with liver cancer. I was happy that he and I were able to speak several times before his death in 2005."

As the Diamond Headache Clinic grew, Seymour increased the size of his physician staff to manage the ever-growing caseload. Some provided a significant boost to the clinic's effectiveness; some did not.

Jose Medina

One of the first associates was Jose Medina, a resident at the Mount Sinai Hospital in neurology whom Seymour met in 1974. Medina was originally from Spain, and he was very interested in learning more about headache treatment. His chief of neurology at the time asked him if he'd like to spend three months studying at the Diamond Headache Clinic, and he jumped at the opportunity. Near the end of his study period, Seymour had a word with him.

"We talked, and he expressed a desire to do more with headache, so I asked him if he'd like to join the practice. However, he and his wife were returning to Spain, but I told him to keep in touch. When they returned, Dr. Medina joined me in practice in 1976. He remained with me for five years.

"With Dr. Medina and his inquisitive and original thoughts, I enjoyed some of my most prolific years in scientific investigation. Together with Frank Rubino, Jose and I published an article in 1975 in the journal *Headache* on patients with transient ischemic attacks. These attacks occur when a patient presents with neurological symptoms for a few seconds or minutes which are related to their headache. We discussed that these attacks did not have dire consequence for the patient.

"Individually, and with Dr. Medina, we published several studies on the use of the drug isometheptene in the abortive therapy of migraine. This medication continues to be used successfully in children and in adults who, for some reason, cannot use triptans or ergot preparations.

"There has been a consistent belief and misconception that allergy had a direct connection to headache. Headache patients were extensively being tested for allergies and unnecessarily being desensitized to a variety of substances. In 1975, I initiated a study on allergy and headache in which we measured the IgE level in migraine patients and that of a comparable group of nonheadache individuals. IgE in the blood is a chemical marker of allergy. We found no differences between the groups. In 1976, Dr. Medina and I published an article, 'Migraine and Atopy,' in the journal *Headache*. During the same year, we published an article on the relationship of sinus disease and headache. This study received little recognition. However, twenty-five years later, with little note of my original work, sinus problems and headache were again the major focus of scientific studies, dissecting any relationship.

"Later in 1976, I published on my groundbreaking study of the beta-blocker propranolol and its use in migraine prophylaxis. [This research is discussed earlier in the book.] Propranolol remains the drug of choice by knowledgeable clinicians to prevent migraine attacks. We conducted research on other beta-blockers and continued to publish our findings. One study was on the alpha blocker clonidine, which demonstrated efficacy in migraineurs with and without hypertension. Although not approved for the indication of migraine prevention, clonidine serves as an option for migraine prophylactic treatment.

"In one of my earlier studies on migraine, I wrote that certain patients experienced a clustering of their migraine attacks with episodes occurring almost daily or multiple attacks reported for a distinct period of time. In this paper, I documented a group of these patients being successfully treated with lithium carbonate. This drug had previously been used effectively for chronic cluster headaches and manic depressive episodes. In 1981, Dr. Medina and I published the article 'Cyclical Migraine' in *Archives of Neurology*.

"I was saddened when Dr. Medina left our practice, but that's life. Jose wanted to practice general neurology. However, he did not continue to do the research that marked his career at the Diamond Headache Clinic.

"After Dr. Medina started his own neurology practice, it was evident that I needed another physician to assist me in the ever-growing practice. I had met a young neurologist at one of my lectures. Although he had only been in practice for about four or five years, he wanted to switch gears and focus on one malady. He was an intelligent young man with a wonderful personality. His patients liked him, and he was also happy to participate in the research that was ongoing at the clinic, including our review of long-term propranolol therapy.

"In 1983, we concurred that we should add another physician, and that was when Fred Freitag joined the staff. Fred was a graduate of Chicago College of Osteopathic Medicine (now Midwestern University) and during his residency had completed a clerkship at Cleveland Clinic under my good friend Bob Kunkel. Fred was very personable, and I noted that he had joined AASH as a resident and had attended a few courses and our annual meetings. He was definitely interested in headache. I also liked the fact that he had completed a residency in family practice.

"Now I had two young physicians assisting me with the practice, as well as research and writing. Then I noticed that our neurologist was becoming lethargic. He wasn't returning patient phone calls, he wasn't meeting deadlines for the research, and his demeanor towards me had changed. I regretfully realized that he was not an asset to the practice, and I asked him to resign. He joined a practice with a chiropractor, focusing on personal injury cases. And sadly, a few years later, I learned that he had committed suicide.

Frederick Freitag

According to his biography on the National Headache Foundation's website, Dr. Freitag received his bachelor of science in biochemistry from the University of Wisconsin and his D.O. degree from the Chicago College of Osteopathic Medicine in 1979. His residency in family medicine was coupled with additional training in headache medicine at the Cleveland Clinic Foundation in 1981. He is certified in family medicine and holds a certificate of added qualification in headache management from the National Board for Certification in Headache Management. He is one of only 290 physicians who have subspecialty certification for headache medicine from the United Council for Neurologic Subspecialties. He is a fellow of the American Headache Society.

"I first heard of Seymour Diamond in 1964," Dr. Freitag remembers. "My best friend in grade school had headaches, and Dr. Diamond's name came up, although that had nothing to do with my decision to pursue headache treatment later in life."

It was Dr. Freitag's medical school experiences that influenced him. "I saw how poorly headache patients were treated, and that's what made me want to focus on headache treatment."

In 1977, when studying for his boards, Freitag came across a copy of *Headache*, the journal of the American Association for the Study of Headache. He contacted Seymour and inquired about becoming a member of the organization. Seymour informed him that they'd never had a student member before, but apparently he was intrigued by the young doctor's enthusiasm and ultimately responded by saying, "Send me a letter from your dean and a $15 membership fee."

Dr. Freitag came to work with Seymour in 1983 after working at the clinic as an extern, and the hiring followed when Seymour realized how helpful his extern could be as a full-time clinic physician.

"Fred was an enthusiastic partner in research and writing," Seymour recalls. "In his first year, we reviewed the use of the beta-blocker nadolol in migraine. With other staff physicians and residents, we published several articles each year on our research, including our work with Aron Mosnaim, Ph.D. Through Dr. Mosnaim's lab at Chicago Medical School, we looked at plasma and platelet methionine-enkephalin levels in our clinic patients. We published studies regarding inpatient care of headaches, with the unit then located at Weiss Memorial Hospital in Chicago. The British Migraine Trust sponsored an international headache congress every two years in London. For each of those meetings, Fred and I would submit several papers for platform and poster presentations. Once accepted, we would then develop manuscripts, which were published in a book detailing the proceedings of the congress. There were several editions of *Advances in Headache Research,* and *New Advances in Headache Research,* edited by my good friend Dr. F. Clifford Rose, which included our work.

"In the years we worked together," Dr. Freitag continues, "I had fewer fights with Seymour than I did with my wife. Seymour revolutionized the field of headache on so many fronts. He put headache on the map."

It is no doubt significant that Dr. Freitag left the Diamond Headache Clinic to launch his own headache clinic when Seymour retired, selling his interest in the Diamond Headache Clinic to his partners. When Dr. Freitag left, he moved to Texas and Baylor University, where he became the medical director of the Comprehensive Headache Center and director of headache medicine research for Baylor Health Care System in Dallas in the fall of 2010, establishing a comprehensive inpatient program in addition to his other responsibilities.

"It was an honor and a pleasure to work with Seymour through the years," Dr. Freitag summarizes, "and because of that, I've been able to move out on my own."

Jordan Prager

Jordan Prager, M.D., joined the Diamond Headache Clinic staff in 1984 after finishing his residency in neurology. "He was a wonderful asset to the clinic—enthusiastic and personable." But after only one year, Jordan realized he didn't like the pace of a busy practice and was looking forward to getting married and starting a family. He was accepted into a radiology residency, and now uses his skills as a neuroradiologist in the NorthShore University HealthSystem in Evanston, Illinois.

Lawrence Robbins, M.D.

After Dr. Prager left, neurologist Lawrence Robbins joined the staff. Seymour notes, "Larry was probably one of the brightest physicians who worked for me—academically bright. He took copious notes on how I treated patients. As an aside, he was also a nationally recognized bridge player."

But after eighteen months, he decided that he had learned enough to start his own practice in the northern suburbs. Dr. Robbins has maintained his headache practice as well as his keen interest in research. He has written several books and utilizes the techniques learned from Seymour at the Diamond Headache Clinic.

Glen Solomon

In 1986, Glen Solomon joined the Diamond Headache Clinic staff following his service in the United States Air Force. Seymour remembers Glen as "a very eager physician."

"Before Glen joined our staff, he had published on his work with the calcium channel blockers in migraine. It was great to add a physician who had headache and research experience," Seymour recalls. Dr. Solomon picked up Seymour's methods quickly and served as a valuable member of the staff for several years.

"During his tenure at the clinic, Glen, Fred, and I published our research with long-acting propranolol in migraine treatment, as well as the NSAIDs and antidepressants in headache therapy. With Glen and Fred, we contributed chapters to a few textbooks, including *Handbook of Chronic Pain Management* (1989) and *Sports Neurology* (1989)."

Dr. Solomon was anxious to leave the Chicago area and took a position at the Cleveland Clinic, working with Dr. Robert Kunkel. He has continued his research activities and is now located at the medical school at Wright State University in Dayton, Ohio, near where he served in the Air Force.

"He was very upright," Seymour recalls and goes on to say that he believes Dr. Solomon continues the techniques that he learned at the Diamond Headache Clinic. With Dr. Merle Diamond, Glen edited the sixth edition of *Diamond and Dalessio's Practicing Physician's Approach to Headache* (1999).

George Urban

Dr. George Urban works at the Diamond Headache Clinic today, more than twenty years after he first approached Seymour in search of a position with the clinic. Seymour recalls hiring him:

"Nice personality with a marked Slovakian accent," Seymour says. "Very intelligent, very warm, the type of person you'd want to take care of people. The only trouble was, a lot of people had trouble understanding him. I liked him very much, but I said, 'George, I'm going to send you to Northwestern. They offer an excellent speech therapy program. I'll pay and let them try to straighten out your speech.' He was fine with that. He wanted the job. It only helped slightly, but patients liked him. He's a good headache doctor."

Dr. Urban currently serves as co-director at the Diamond Headache Clinic. His bio is posted on the clinic's website along with a quote by Dr. Urban:

"First visit is always stressful. I try to break down the barrier so the patient feels comfortable and reduces their stress level. I ask what their expectation is, and if it's a cure, I tell them right away, we don't do that. I tell them what they can have is a better life with reduced frequency and severity so they can get back to doing what they want."

According to the Diamond Headache Clinic website, "Dr. Urban is a native of Presov, Czechoslovakia. He graduated from Safarik University Medical School in 1974, and from there, completed a residency and fellowship in Neurology at the Municipal Hospital, Kosice, Czechoslovakia. Dr. Urban came to the United States in 1985, first settling in San Francisco, and then moving to the Midwest to pursue a residency in Internal Medicine at Rosalind Franklin University of Medicine and Science in Chicago.

"He joined the staff of the Diamond Headache Clinic in 1990, and since has taken a strong interest in the treatment of headache with BOTOX injections. He is currently on the staff of Saint Joseph Hospital and is a Clinical Instructor, Department of Medicine, at Rosalind Franklin University of Medicine and Science, and a Lecturer, Department of Medicine (Neurology), Loyola University Chicago/Stritch School of Medicine.

"[Dr. Urban] has lectured on various headache subjects throughout his career, and is actively conducting research at the clinic."

Bernard Shulman

"We were in medical school about the same time," Dr. Bernard Shulman, now retired, recalls. "I'm a couple of years older than he is, but I first met him when we were both in medical school. Then years later, when St. Joseph's hospital opened up, we were both at the hospital. I was the head of psychiatry, and Seymour had a practice specializing in headache. I became the psychiatrist for his patients, and he became my headache man.

"That's how we met and got together. Some of us in the hospital would get together socially, and Seymour was one of them.

"I thought he was interesting. He was trying to do something special, something that was needed. I felt that he knew what he was doing, and eventually, he was bringing his patients into the hospital. I was informed that Seymour wanted to bring some of his patients into the hospital and put them in the new psychiatric unit that we had, which was okay with me, but not okay with somebody in administration. They felt he couldn't put his patients on the psychiatric unit without having somebody else come in. So then Seymour opened up a unit at another hospital.

"Seymour asked me to help him with what he was trying to do. He was creating an organization and began to bring out his own journal. And he was building up a headache program at the hospital, which became international. He was getting patients from all over, from England, for example, and also other countries. The journal was a good journal, and he was able to build the headache program, the American Association for the Study of Headache.

"When he published his books and the journal, if there was some psychiatric issue, he would ask me to write something for him. So, I helped him with his publications, too.

"About twenty years after that, I ended my position as head of the department at St. Joseph's Hospital, and he invited me to come and work at the hospital where he was at the time.

"They had a whole unit—a headache unit—and it was the first time I had seen the way he put things together in his unit. I performed the duty of psychiatrist, and they also employed a psychologist.

"I worked with Seymour for about another twenty years. He did something that was new and was good and helpful, and he had a lot of patients, and patients liked working with him. On the national scene, he was president of the society which, really, he had created, and tried to spread what he was doing.

"In my opinion, he was very successful in what he was doing. He'd done things nobody else had thought of. And Seymour himself was a likable guy. He was able to attract people that would support his program, and he still has the association. I'm still a member of it, although I can't get there anymore.

"We always had psychologists because Seymour was using all sorts of techniques. I applied some of the techniques and supported it. And he had a program, not using medication, but using biofeedback.

"If something was new to the market or if someone had a new idea, Seymour immediately tried to do something with it. And he had an awful lot of interesting patients. And we did a good job!

"I think of Seymour as somebody that made a real contribution to American medicine, to the whole world of medicine that was centered around headache, but headache mixed in with other things.

"We socialized. Neither one of us was a drinker, but we both enjoyed a good meal. Our professional interests were very close, and we tried to help each other where we could be of some use.

"Actually, as he was building his program, I was building my own program. He was a success. I was a success also. I was able to build a school for psychologists, the Adler School of Professional Psychology in Chicago. So, in that particular sense, we were two successful people.

"We never had an argument. Never. I never saw him do anything that I would find fault with, and I don't think he found fault in what I did. I would take the patients and take the nurses and the students—we always had students from someplace—and have them work with me. It created a friendly atmosphere in the unit. The people who were working there liked it.

"Most of the time, the patients liked us, too!" Dr. Shulman concluded with a laugh.

Robert Kunkel

Another longtime associate and good friend is Dr. Robert Kunkel, who shows up in Seymour's history in the early 1970s. The National Headache Foundation's website offered this biographical sketch:

> Dr. Robert Kunkel, a member of the Cleveland Clinic Foundation (CCF) staff, has served in a number of capacities since 1960, when he joined CCF as an intern staff physician. Since that time he has devoted his energies to the headache sufferer and is currently maintaining his practice (editor's note: Dr. Kunkel has retired now), as well as acting as a consultant for the Section of Headache in the CCF Department of Neurology. Not only has he been a member of the NHF Board of Directors since 1983, but he served as its President for eleven years. He received the National Migraine Foundation Lectureship Award in 1985 and the Patient Partners Award in 2002. Dr. Kunkel enjoys the ice sport of curling.

Dr. Kunkel joined the Cleveland Clinic as an intern in 1960, completing his residency in internal medicine. He served in the U.S. Army as a doctor stationed in Alaska before returning to Cleveland Clinic as a staff physician in the Sections of Headache in both the Department of Internal Medicine and the Department of Neurology.

Dr. Kunkel was with Seymour during the campaign that concluded with his "beheading," or expulsion, from the American Association for the Study of Headache.

"Seymour was one of the most important people in getting headache recognized as a legitimate health concern," Dr. Kunkel recalls, "but we were all not neurologists, so a lot of us—particularly Seymour in his leadership role—were not accepted by a lot of neurology people. Some of us who were not neurologists stuck together because we were frowned upon by the neurologists.

"I think there were several younger neurologists who were getting interested in headache and felt that Seymour was keeping them out of the organization. At that time, he was the executive director of the organization. He had served as president and his sister Idell was running the meetings, so really Seymour and his office ran things. And that's what caused some of the conflicts. Some of the younger people wanted more of a voice within the organization. They felt that too much control was with Seymour, and that's what led to his being asked to step down as executive director.

"I can see the other side of it. Seymour, as you know, is a general practitioner, and they felt that headache was a neurological disorder, so therefore, they should be more involved with this organization. They felt that it was time for 'other people' to take the leadership role.

"It was a real sticky time because Seymour had done so much to get the association going. He really made it what it was, and yet these other people felt that they couldn't participate, that they were being locked out, if you will. It was a sad time."

When Seymour left AASH, the National Migraine Foundation he'd created left with him, evolving into today's National Headache Foundation, and Dr. Kunkel was an active supporter from the beginning.

"I'm an emeritus board member," he says today. "I stepped down from being an active board member a couple of years ago. Having been on it for thirtysome years, I felt it was time to step aside and let some younger people come on the board."

Dr. Kunkel and his wife, Brenda, became good friends with Seymour and Elaine, often traveling together around the world for medical conferences and enjoying the discoveries offered by the various cultures.

Seymour has been criticized for his driving abilities, and driving abroad provided even more challenges.

"I'm not sure when it was ... " Dr. Kunkel begins. "'85 or '86 maybe. We met in London every other year with the headache work group of the World Federation of Neurology. And one year, the Diamonds and we went to Ireland after the London meeting, and we had a little minivan.

"We joke about him scraping all the paint off the side of the van because of all those narrow roads in Ireland with the hedgerows, and he's driving on the other side of the road, of course. At first, we'd take turns driving, but Elaine finally felt that it would be best if I drove all the time. Seymour gets impatient at times, and we often had to sit and wait for sheep wandering out in the road."

Concerning Seymour's contributions to headache medicine, Dr. Kunkel says, "He was probably the most important person in the field of headache back in the late '60s, early '70s. And, again, for a person who wasn't a neurologist … as I've said, that was a problem because a lot of people didn't really accept him, but for the headache patient, he certainly was a great man. He had promoted the fact that headache is a real, legitimate medical problem and not all psychiatric, as everybody thought back then."

Alex Feoktistov

In Moscow, Russia, in the year 2001, a young neurologist dreamed what seemed like an impossible dream. Alex Feoktistov had completed his initial medical education in neurology and then he added a Ph.D. in headache study to his string of postname initials. Now what?

"Back in Russia I did my residency in neurology, and after that I did the Ph.D. training in headaches, over there in Moscow. And we had this special school called The Presidential Stipend—a presidential grant for one year of research abroad, the Yeltsin Award. It's a competition for fifty grants for research outside. And it wasn't just for medicine. It was for futuristic projects in medicine, physics, or mathematics.

"I applied for this program, and it took a year probably to go through this whole competition process. And I was lucky enough to win one of those. The concept was fairly simple; they basically said they were going to sponsor you for one year of research, but it's your responsibility to find the place where you want to go.

"The Diamond Headache Clinic was my first choice because I was studying headache and … in particular, medication for chronic headaches and chronic migraines.

"So I wanted to come here, but I sent my resume to different places, including Diamond Headache Clinic. Then, once I had sent my resume, the people in Russia—the ones who were running this whole competition process—they said, 'You have only one week to get a reply. Otherwise, we will send somebody else. So you need to find the place where you want to go in one week!' Nobody told us about this ahead of time.

"I had sent applications to twenty different places, twenty different clinics all over the world. Most of them were in the United States. There were a few in Canada, a few in Germany, and a few in Italy.

"Dr. Diamond replied first, and I still remember that night—it was one o'clock in the morning. My fax machine started making the funny noises, and I lifted the fax and it was the letter from Dr. Diamond saying that they accepted me! That was the quickest reply that our department had ever seen. A lot of people that I talked to who had entered the same program said sometimes it takes you a month just to get a reply. That's why we were skeptical that I would be able to go because one week was just not realistic.

"It was an unbelievable feeling when he replied in three days. On that third day we got a fax with all the expenses and everything that needed to be done, all the formalities. So, I basically got all the papers ready, and that's how we came here. It was November 23, 2001."

Dr. Feoktistov's dream quickly became a reality. He and his wife Elena (who is a cardiologist) flew into Chicago and almost immediately, he met with the renowned Dr. Diamond.

"We flew in, and my wife and I went for a walk. It was rainy weather. It was kind of coldish, and we went to a lake, which was in the neighborhood in Lincoln Park not too far from the clinic. I had an appointment with him scheduled in the morning, I think at 8:00 a.m. at his office. Night and day. So we got no transition whatsoever. We basically came in and went straight ahead.

"I remember I was surprised at that. In Russia, we have physicians who would start work early, and they would make appointments at such an early time, but I didn't expect it to occur so fast.

"Anyway, I walked into the clinic, and I was introduced to Dr. Diamond. My first impression was that he was very easy to talk to.

That was my first time outside Russia and there, when a person is famous, you they are often difficult to approach. You have to schedule things, and they'd rather you talk to their associates or assistants and not to the person himself. But here, this man was sitting there himself. Very, very approachable, and very nice, very kind, very straightforward in his thoughts. So that was a nice, unexpected impression. I was thrilled and relieved at the same time!

"I didn't start seeing patients that day with him—I just made the rounds, you know, they showed me around the clinic, explained to me how the clinic is working, and what was done in the clinic, so I could get an idea of the flow of how things are done.

"And also another thing, actually, I forgot to mention what overimpressed me: I used to work in the first Moscow Headache Clinic for probably six months prior to coming here. It was a very modern clinic, very European, and we had couple of new treatment approaches over there. So I brought some brochures with me to show him what kind of clinic we had over there.

"In comparison, the Diamond Headache Clinic was huge and very well developed with a longstanding tradition of headache treatment. But I'd brought those brochures with me with the information about the Moscow Clinic, and he actually looked at them, and then he asked one of his associates to go through it and see if there's anything that they can incorporate into their clinic here. I was very surprised! It was very unusual. He was open-minded and not shy at all as far as learning something new.

"I think next morning I met him again in the hospital for rounds, and that was another positive impression. I still remember. I keep telling everybody—all my friends and family just compared from when I was in Moscow, my Moscow boss who was the head of the neurology department, Professor Vein. He was a very famous neurologist and one of the smartest people I'd ever seen in my life. He was my real hero idol, I guess, when I was studying neurology back in Moscow.

"But with all that respect and everything, I still felt like he was not as easily approachable as Dr. Diamond. I remember we were working with him, and one of the patients approached Professor Vein and asked him some questions about the treatment or something, but he'd never seen this patient before and she was referred to him. But, usually, what they do in Russia when they refer someone for Professor Vein's consultation, they need to go to his department and one of his associates will see you. Not necessarily him in person.

"That was a very common approach in Russia. When I came here, I remember working with Dr. Diamond in the hospital. And one time a patient stopped him in the hallway to ask him a couple of things about her treatment. She was a patient of one of the other doctors, and she was just concerned about some side effects. He talked to her and explained, and then he looked down at the chart, and he talked to the nurse to make a couple of changes. And I was also surprised that he was so open-minded, and he was so easy to deal with, even with patients.

"All these impressions were emphasized during later years when I saw him with patients, and talking to them, and how he was treating them. His approach was what I probably would call 'old school.' He doesn't just rely on the imaging. He doesn't just rely on the medication. He actually talks to the patient. He spends time, especially with new patients, and it's different. Even these days, even in this country, I don't think there are too many doctors who have that same humanlike approach to the patients."

Seymour firmly believes in medical education, and helping an enthusiastic young doctor who seemed to have the same level of interest in headache medicine as he himself probably came as second nature. He offered not only advice and hands-on training, but he also encouraged Dr. Feoktistov's natural curiosity and interest in research.

"Since I came for research essentially, I wanted to do some research in chronic daily headache, and Dr. Diamond gave me an idea. He said, 'We have this inpatient facility here. Why don't you try to do something with that?" I wanted to investigate the inpatient efficacy, or the inpatient treatment, of patients with intractable chronic daily headaches.

"I made a plan and explained it to him, what I think might be interesting to do and how to investigate, which parameters we should analyze. He approved everything, and we started doing the study where I would be coming to the hospital every day, talking to patients, writing everything down in my Excel file on my computer, and then analyzing it.

"By the end of the year, I showed him the results, and it was a success. Basically it proved that inpatient treatment was successful for patients who did not benefit from the outpatient treatment previously. So he was very excited about that. And then, the month we completed the study, we published it, we sent it for a poster, and it was accepted in Italy for the International Headache Society meeting for a poster presentation. Dr. Diamond didn't feel like going there, so I didn't go, either. I just wanted to finish my work here."

Dr. Feoktistov was only scheduled to be in America on his research/study junket for a limited amount of time. He was obligated to return to Russia unless something else happened. Luckily, it did.

"I remember I was sitting in his office in the hospital (Dr. Feoktistovalso had an office in the hospital), and I asked him about extending my program here because it was the end of my year. And I felt I did a good start, and I was thinking maybe we should expand it a little bit.

"I also like the American lifestyle, the way the medicine works here; it was very different from Russia. I guess I was thinking about maybe staying here. Even if it meant staying here temporarily for a little bit longer than that year. Initially, it was a ten-month program.

"So, I remember that he was sitting in front of me, he smiled, and he said, 'Would you like to join my clinic in the future?'

"I said, 'Of course!' and added that it was my dream job. It's one of the best clinics in the world, if not *the* best, as far as headache goes. So I said, 'Of course, I'd love to sometime in the future when I have my license and everything is in order. Sure, that would be great. It would be a dream come true.'

"He smiled and said, 'I'd like you to join my clinic once we have that opportunity.'

"Back then I didn't even know what I needed to do to get a medical license because I never thought about it, about staying in this country. We essentially came just for this ten months' research. So I didn't have any information about what it takes, which tests I needed to do. I knew nothing.

"Neither did he, I think. So he called one of his friends that was somehow involved in this education process and asked. I remember just sitting and talking with him about this and thinking that in Russia, you ask about something like this and people say, 'Okay, we'll schedule an appointment, we'll call …' and then maybe a couple of weeks later they may. If you're lucky, you can get some information back.

"But he just picked up the phone and called right away. To somebody, to one of his friends and just asked him, in very simple words, what needs to be done. 'I have this kid sitting in front of me. He wants to get a medical license. What does he need to do?' And they explained to him in just a few words. And he told me what needed to be done.

"And then, from that time on, he supported me 120 percent. All of my efforts, all of my time. You know, because I was working, I was studying for my board examination, to get into the residency. So he helped me significantly.

"He was like my father here. He was my family here. He was helping me and my family in every way possible. And I felt that support all the time, *all the time*, which was also very unusual. We kind of bonded from the first day."

As it turns out, Seymour created a new training method to use with Dr. Feoktistov that was an improvement on his earlier processes. With earlier trainees, he'd looked at their patients' charts and then quizzed the trainee on his or her decisions. He feels the new method, as described here by Dr. Feoktistov, is more effective.

"Another thing about my time with him: I wasn't just following him around and seeing how he talks to the patients, how he treats them, and what his treatment philosophy was. What he asked me to do—and I'm really, really thankful for that—every time he would see new patients, he would send me into the room to talk to the patients first, and I would get all the information, all the history. I would write everything down. I wasn't able to sign anything obviously because I didn't have my license. But I would just do all the paperwork, including the patient's history, complaints, and everything. And that's what's important to make the diagnosis.

"And then, on a separate piece of paper, he had me write the diagnosis—what I think it is—and then my treatment and diagnosis plan.

"I would do that for every single new patient, and then I'd leave the patient for a few moments to talk with him. He'd be waiting outside the room for me, and he would ask me to present the case to him. So, I presented the case and explained what's going on with this patient and all that, about his headaches. And then he would ask what I think the diagnosis is. I'd tell him the diagnosis, actually—no, he wouldn't ask me—he would just get this information. And then he would walk with me into the room to see the patient himself.

"Without looking at my notes or anything, he would ask the patient a few more questions. And then he would just—it was funny—he would just extend his arm towards me with his palm up and say, 'Give me your list, and let's see what you wrote there.'

"I'd give him my piece of paper, he would look at it, and he would say that he agreed or not, and then he would sign off on it and say, 'Okay, that's right.'

"He would actually give me the clues right away as to whether I was right or I was wrong. And I think that as the time went by, I was more often right than I was wrong with his patients.

"It's been what, ten years? Over nine years since I first came here, and now I'm practicing in the Diamond Headache Clinic. And I use the exact same approach as he used ten years ago. I didn't really change anything I did, and I was surprised that it stuck in my mind so firmly."

Although Dr. Feoktistov is indeed a staff physician at the Diamond Headache Clinic today, he first had to acquire his medical license and complete his education.

"I went away for four years to do the internal medicine residency program. I finally took my boards, my United States Medical License Examination. I passed all of those, and I got into the residency training program in Chicago, right in the same hospital where the Diamond Headache Clinic has its inpatient unit.

"We stayed in touch all those years; we would call each other once in a while for holidays. And then, I was on my third year of residence, and he called me to ask me about my plans in the future, whether I wanted to come back.

"I wanted to, but I also wanted to do a fellowship as well. I thought that could help me as a professional, and he supported me on that and said, 'Sure, that sounds like something that you probably want to do.'

"So then, after completing my internal medicine residency program, I went for one year of the pain management fellowship training program at the Cleveland Clinic.

"He also called me during my fellowship. We stayed in touch, and we talked to each other quite often. And then I think before the end of my fellowship, he called me again and asked, 'So what are your plans now?'

"I said 'If you have an opportunity, I'd like to … I'm open to … I'm looking for a job right now …' because I didn't feel comfortable. I knew where I wanted to go. I knew that I wanted to come here [to the Diamond Headache Clinic], but I didn't know whether he had an opening. And I didn't feel comfortable pushing myself into the clinic. I'd rather come here comfortably than just, you know, running into it.

"But he said, 'I think there's a good opportunity. We have a couple of positions retired, if you're open to that …'

"I didn't want even to hear anything else. I said, 'Yes! I'll do that! I'll come for an interview.' I had my mind set that I wanted to be part of it. I just waited for a good opportunity, so I interviewed for a staff position. I didn't have an interview with him this time; it was with his daughter, who is director of the clinic now.

"Another thing that also impressed me was that he was very sharp and had strict views on how to run the clinic. I knew that he wanted things to be done in a certain way, and he had the right because he created the whole clinic, so he knew what worked and what didn't.

"At the same time, he remained very energetic, funny at times, *human*. He was not kind of—how do I put it—he didn't live in extremes. He wasn't just an all business person and nothing is funny in life. He works very hard, harder than I've ever seen people working, and at the same time, he knows how to enjoy life. He knows how to socialize and make things fun.

"He was very strict, and if things didn't go right, he would let you have it! With me, I think he was very kind. He would just say, 'I don't think so,' or something very simple, and the discussion would end at that point. I don't remember him having any hard issues. I've never actually seen him yell. I've seen him being frustrated or upset about things, but it just would be … emotionally he would get upset, but I don't think he would ever yell at somebody.

"It was his attitude, the words he would use. He would tell you that this is not the way it's supposed to be done. Things need to be changed. But at the same time, he would be very polite and professional."

Seymour says the following of Dr. Feoktistov: "He spent almost six years with me. If there's anybody who knows my method, or my art, of treating headache patients, he knows it. And one of the reasons is the way I trained him. I would have him go in and see a patient and do a history and a physical and neurological exam, and then I would insist that he write down his diagnosis and his course of treatment.

"I always took new doctors in with me to show them how to build a relationship with patients," Seymour continues. "I told them that they should always know something personal about the patient, his origin, occupation, hobbies, or something about the person that shows that you appreciate him or her as an individual.

"One day, I was initiating Dr. George Nissan, a recent addition to the clinic, in the patient interview. Dr. Feoktistov was with us. I went in to see a patient on a return visit, and I asked the patient how he was feeling. I shook his hand, and then said to Dr. Nissan and Dr. Feoktistov, 'This man comes from Dixon, Illinois. Do you know why Dixon, Illinois, is important?'"

Neither doctor spoke. Seymour knows that Dixon, Illinois, is the boyhood home of former U.S. President Ronald Reagan, but he wasn't about to give away the answer. So he offered a hint: "Who solved the Cold War?"

"Immediately, Dr. Feoktistov piped up and said, 'Gorbachev!'" Seymour laughs. "I guess his history books were different than ours."

Clealand Baker

In June 1973, at the annual meeting of the American Association for the Study of Headache at the Plaza Hotel in New York, Seymour delivered the Presidential Address, a lecture discussing research in migraine treatments and the Food and Drug Administration's policies on approving new drugs for headache.

"Within the talk, I offered some criticisms of the Food and Drug Administration, its attitude toward medicine that might be helpful to headache sufferers, and its overregulation, which was improper and destructive in my thoughts.

"After I finished the talk, a short, dignified man, who at that time was VP of legal affairs for a company known as Burroughs Wellcome, came up and introduced himself and congratulated me on my talk. His name was Clealand Baker, and he especially liked the fact that I brought in some political factors that were apropos to the problems that existed with headache medicine.

"Over the years, we became very close friends. In fact, when I lectured in North Carolina, I lectured before his company, and I stayed at his home. When my daughter Merle was applying to Duke, she stayed there, too.

"At that time, we [NHF] didn't feel we wanted board members who were affiliated with a drug company. But when he retired, I asked him to join the foundation's board. And he was one of the brightest idea men I'd ever dealt with.

"In my personal discussions with him, I discussed the issue that doctors treating headache patients were having difficulty in getting reimbursement. At this stage, the majority of patients seen were insured, but insurance companies either gave minimal reimbursement or none at all for headache.

"In my conversations with Clea, I also mentioned the fact that there was no standard methodology in the treatment of headache patients. It was varied and unorganized, differing from doctor to doctor.

"At that point, I established a committee to originate a standards of care document. We hired a writer and went to work."

The finished work was originally published in the *Cleveland Clinic Journal*. Today, it's available as a 181-page booklet called *Standards of*

Care for Headache Diagnosis and Treatment to health care practitioners from the National Headache Foundation.

What's actually in the booklet? A lot, but an overview of the document suitable for laypeople can be found on the National Headache Foundation's website at headaches.org.

Seymour's friend and idea man Clealand Baker came up with the brainstorm to create a certificate of added qualification. The group set up criteria and requirements which, when met, would result in the certificate being awarded to headache doctors. Further, they created a committee of headache doctors from around the U.S., as Seymour calls them, "the movers and shakers" of headache medicine.

Then, when an insurance company denied coverage on a headache-related diagnosis or treatment, a letter explaining the need for the coverage along with a copy of the standards of care would be provided to them. A measure of persuasive conversation was added when necessary.

It took time, but eventually headache medicine and treatments became understood and accepted, and it was the National Headache Foundation's standards of care document that paved the way for well-treated patients and happily reimbursed doctors.

Clealand Baker died on March 15, 2008, only two weeks after Jene, his wife of sixty-eight years passed away. She was ninety-three and he, ninety-two.

"Clea Baker was a longtime NHF board member whose imagination and creativity helped the foundation to reach its ultimate goal of service to the headache sufferer," Seymour said after his friend's death. "I considered him a close friend and confidante, and he is missed by one and all."

Roger Cady

From the Headachecare.com website: "Dr. [Roger] Cady is the founder of Headache Care Center, Clinvest, and Primary Care Education.

"He is a graduate of the Mayo Medical School, and is Board Certified by the American Board of Family Practice. . . . He was the co-recipient of the prestigious Wolff Award in 2000 from the American Headache Society for his research entitled 'The Spectrum of Headache.' Dr. Cady is associate executive director at the National Headache Foundation."

Seymour has officially retired from the Diamond Headache Clinic, but he continues to work as executive chairman for the National Headache Foundation. Dr. Cady has been an enthusiastic participant in the NHF as well as in his research and practice, and Seymour expects that when he finally retires completely, Dr. Cady will be his likely successor to lead the NHF.

"I think it's fair to say that I knew Dr. Diamond long before I met him," Dr. Cady begins. "I think the very first time I actually met him was at an investigator meeting for a drug called sumatriptan (Imitrex). It was my very first time doing a large and very important clinical trial, and of course, he was one of the icons whose books I'd read, whose name I recognized, and whose reputation I admired. I think that was the very first time we met.

"I doubt he even remembered me or [remembered] that I was there, but it was through that effort that I got connected a little bit, and then I joined the NHF, and in a way started establishing my own credibility.

"The truth was, I'm kind of a bit of an odd egg in the headache community in that I'm a family physician. So is Dr. Diamond, and by and large, the field of headache is populated by neurologists. So, I think that was an immediate connection between us—a real focus on the patient side of headache rather than just the academic side of headache.

"As it turned out, I became the first doctor involved in that important step of introducing brand-new treatments for migraine, which was sumatriptan. After I published my study, that's probably when Seymour and I became better connected. I was a newcomer in this field with a different background than many of the other physicians. I still appreciate how supporting he was with my pursuing headache as a professional specialty.

"I think the most important lesson I learned from Seymour involves his focus on patients. There's a whole academic side to the field of headache, and that's important. But he focused on the quality of patient care, the ability to communicate and understand the patient. And I think more than anything—and his scientific contributions go without saying—there were so few people that really focused on the quality of care from the patient's perspective. So, I think more than anything, that's what I remember. I remember in the context of lectures he would give, many personal conversations—we'd shared patients at times over the years—and I just think the quality and the ability for him to connect and learn from and help patients ... that, to me, is the most incredible thing.

"A lot of people have done academic medicine well, and Seymour is certainly at the top of that list. But that focus on patients was critical.

"In my mind, and I think in the minds of most others, Seymour Diamond is the father of modern-day headache.

"Headache was sort of an orphaned disease. Certainly that was its state when Dr. Diamond started. And he really did a lot to mainstream it and to validate headache as a real and important medical disease," Dr. Cady concludes.

Seymour has chosen Dr. Cady to succeed him as leader of the National Headache Foundation not only because of his headache expertise, but also because he considers him to be "a good, aggressive businessman." That assignation occurred when Seymour hired a consultant to advise them on the NHF's future, and the consultant informed them that the organization had no "pattern of succession." The only problem, as Seymour saw when he announced his intentions to have Dr. Cady replace him, was that people seemed to think he was going to quit on the spot! Of course, he had only laid the plan for Dr. Cady to take over when Seymour eventually decides he's no longer able to continue himself.

Richard Hawkins

Seymour met Dr. Richard Hawkins at a Chicago Medical School Alumni Association reunion. Hawkins was president of Finch University (now Rosalind Franklin University, where the Chicago Medical School is located) at the time, and he remembers an incident in which Seymour's influence was beneficial, but in an embarrassing way, to one of the school's administrators.

"It's sort of a cute story," Dr. Hawkins begins. "Seymour and I met casually through the Chicago Medical School Alumni Association. I found him very astute. And one time, we wanted to invite Sir John Vane to speak at the medical school. Vane had won the Nobel Prize for Physiology [or Medicine] in 1982, and so we wanted to invite him in to speak. One of the vice presidents said he knew him, and he was telling our board chairman Mr. Finch, 'We should invite this man to be a distinguished lecturer.' Well, as it turned out later, he had to confess that Vane wouldn't answer his telephone calls!

"So I waited. I talked to Seymour about it, and he told me he had invited Dr. Vane to the U.S. to receive an award from the National Headache Foundation and that he had accepted the invitation. So, when everybody was together, I asked Mr. Finch if he'd like to have John Vane as a speaker. I told him I could arrange it through Seymour Diamond. And the vice president who'd failed at recruiting Dr. Vane almost fell off his chair!

"So, that's how it evolved. We began to work together on various issues. Seymour needed accreditation for some of his CME (continuing medical education) programs, and I helped him with that. Then I wanted to get some scholarships for the students—or for the alumni—and Seymour helped me get the funding for those.

"You know, the funny thing is, I think many of his colleagues were jealous of his intellectual abilities. As a group, they could be rather small-minded.

"Coming back to Mr. Finch, he didn't really care for Seymour although he was very, very clever about not saying so. 'Well,' he'd say, 'Dr. Diamond … I really don't know much about his practice, but I know that he managed to cure my brother-in-law of headaches that he had all his life and no one else could do it.' He'd give that sort of backhanded compliment.

"Seymour wanted to be on the board of the Chicago Medical School, and I wanted him to be on the board, but we could never arrange that. I think he was just a little too astute for the others. It would have been wonderful if he had joined the board. He could see through a lot of the nonsense that others were bringing to the table.

"The Chicago Medical School Alumni Association was key in Seymour's life. They gave him the Distinguished Alumnus Award in 1977 for his pioneering efforts in diagnosis and treatment of headache."

At the same presentation where Seymour received the Distinguished Alumnus Award, he notes with a grin that another well-known doctor received his acknowledgement as well, albeit posthumously: Dr. William H. Scholl, the name behind Dr. Scholl foot care products.

Seymour also received the Distinguished Alumnus Award from the Chicago Medical School Alumni Association in 2002. The President's Award was presented by the president of the Chicago Medical School Alumni Association, Dr. Eugene Rogers. Dr. Rogers and his wife, Joyce, were also good friends with Seymour and Elaine.

"I very quickly came to realize that he was one of the most famous alumni of the Chicago Medical School!" Dr. Hawkins continues.

"And he was incredibly successful. He combined the business knowledge with the need—people who'd been suffering from headache. It's so debilitating to some that they'd do anything to be relieved of these headaches. He had a very methodical approach. He realized everything that was necessary to not only diagnose but to treat the problem. His approach was to stay with the patient until they'd gone over everything and controlled the headache.

"Seymour's strength was that he'd keep going at it, doggedly searching for a scientific relief—in a very logical way—until he found the answer for that particular patient, whether it was diet, hormonal, or whatever it happened to be. Some of these patients were on many, many medicines and weren't getting any relief from their neurologists. And so they went to Seymour. He became world-famous doing this!

"He's very thorough, a very dedicated man. He's very empathetic, and he brought that to the patients with the science behind it. But then ... well, the empathy, the science ... but in order to run a large clinic, you have to have the wherewithal. He realized he needed a hospital base. He established that with Columbus and then later with St. Joseph's. He was a star there. He had a whole ward filled with headache patients. But he has the vision to see everything that was necessary to help the patient, to really give them relief.

"We were never competitors. He's a medical doctor; I'm a physiologist. I was under administration or teaching or research in different areas. So we found common ground and worked together," Dr. Hawkins concludes.

Arthur Elkind

"I met Seymour about 1968," Dr. Elkind begins. "We met in San Francisco at an American Medical Association meeting. I was from a hospital in the Bronx called Montefiore Medical Center that had a headache clinic. The Headache Clinic at Montefiore was attached to Columbia University Medical School and started probably around 1950 or so. It preceded Seymour's private headache clinic. Montefiore was the first in the country."

Dr. Arnold Friedman had founded Montefiore's Headache Clinic, the first in the U.S. (Seymour's would become the first one operated by a private individual rather than a hospital) and served as its director for almost thirty years.

"Dr. Friedman was very academic," Dr. Elkind continues. "He was ... very proud, a pompous little individual, and he did not have any confidence in the group that Seymour belonged to, the American Headache Society, which at that time, was called the American Association for the Study of Headache.

"He didn't want any of his clinic's physician members to associate with people from the organization. He felt they were not scientific. He was a Harvard graduate, and he was involved with Harvard Medical School. He was very proud of his affiliations, and he felt that the AASH was not very scientific.

"Dr. Friedman told me to be very wary about what I'd hear about their different research and all because he didn't have that much confidence in it. This was in '68. The meeting went on about three or four days, and then finally we spoke—Seymour had a booth right next to us. We had an exhibition, and Seymour had an exhibition.

"Gradually we became friends. And then Dr. Friedman, over the ensuing years, became more relaxed as he grew older. He retired in 1973, and I became the director of the Headache Clinic at Montefiore. He kept in touch, and he still had some contacts with our headache clinic even though he moved to Arizona.

"He gradually softened, and he enjoyed meeting the other people, including Seymour, in the late '70s at different meetings. And he warmed up to the fact they were becoming scientific, that the studies were very substantial. Then, Seymour invited Arnold Friedman into their group. He became a board member, and he became the president, probably in the early '80s.

"Arnold Friedman became very warm towards the group, and then he became involved with the National Headache Foundation. So we all had a very friendly relationship, but it started off on very strange terms.

"Seymour eventually got me into the organization, and I became a board member at large. At the time, I think Arnold became the president. Seymour was the executive director.

"But sometime in the mid-'80s, there were a few ... people on it who were very ambitious, self-destructive, and very difficult to deal with. Basically, it was a group of neurologists who were young people at the time, there to finish their training or a few years after their training. They had this notion that you couldn't treat headache patients unless you were a neurologist, and you certainly couldn't be an executive member of a board of an organization that represented headache professionally. They were obstructionists to physicians who weren't neurologists but who were taking very good care of headache patients. They felt that we were intruding on their territory, even though I did run the headache clinic in Montefiore, one of the most prestigious headache clinics in the country.

"They were very self-centered people, and we had a difficult time dealing with them. Finally, they separated Seymour from the organization at a very disturbing meeting. They had been very friendly to him, and Seymour had befriended some of them and helped them set up their own practices because at that time Seymour's practice was already flourishing in Chicago.

"He helped a group in Michigan and another group in Texas. He helped set up headache clinics, provided practical information and what to do and so forth. But they all turned. They felt that Seymour was taking up too much power in the organization. And there were a lot of perks if you were an administrator in the organization and a physician. There were all kinds of perks in the pharmaceutical companies, advertising firms, etc. These people wanted to get involved, and they didn't want Seymour around. They told him he was no longer executive director. I don't remember exactly how it happened, but there was a board meeting I remember very clearly. They voted Seymour out, and they voted another director in.

"When they did that, they suffered. They sort of cut their throats in several ways. One physician who was an administrator, the head of a department of neurology in Kansas that then moved to Oklahoma, spent huge amounts of money in advertising, but they put something like the wrong date of the meeting on all the publications, and all the mailings that went out were incorrect. But they were very anxious to use their power—it sounds kind of silly in a medical group, but like any other group, it happens.

"They didn't criticize the doctor or anything for his error although he cost the organization a small fortune, and there was a real disturbance in the way the meeting was subsequently set up because the dates were all wrong. Things of this sort happened along with a lot of other things. They raised the dues and did things that were irritating to many board members. Seymour tried to come back and become an active administrator, but they barred him, frankly.

"It was very disturbing to me to have this group of people, who were purportedly his friends, but who then turned on him. In that one meeting his position was taken away, he was voted off the board, and there was a lot of acrimonious discussion at that time, and Seymour was really hurt and insulted. It was a very disturbing meeting.

"After that, Seymour went his way and continued to have instructional courses. I think the physician population enjoyed Seymour's courses a lot more than the headache association's courses, which were run by neurologists. Theirs were more or less academic scientific courses, which was not very helpful for patients, to teach physicians how to treat patients. So the Diamond Headache Clinic courses were much better for physicians who were trying to learn the basics of how to approach a headache patient and take care of him or her.

"Recently, the association did honor him at their annual meeting. They honored him because he was actually one of the original founders of this American Association for the Study of Headache, now called the American Headache Society. Most of the other people had retired and left the field. So, they became friendly to him, some of them, anyway. Some of them are still very cold.

"Seymour made a lot of other friends in the neurology population. It wasn't as if all the neurologists had blackballed him. Actually, a majority of the neurologists who were practicing neurology or doing headache work were very friendly to Seymour.

"It was a very busy, very exciting period at the time when we were actively working."

The glory days of headache?

"Well, it was. But it changed dramatically due to changes in medical remuneration, medical economics, and so forth. The drug companies were doing tremendous research and developing new drugs for headache in the '80s and '90s, up until a few years ago. And then many of the larger companies lost interest in headache as an area to develop new drugs, new treatments, because it wasn't profitable for them—companies like Merck, Pfizer, AstraZeneca, Johnson & Johnson. Although they did have some products, but they were relatively unimportant to them when you look at the global picture for a company like Johnson & Johnson or Pfizer.

"But back then, they each had their own drugs and made a very marked change in treatment of headache patients. Now the new drugs that are coming out are really byproducts of what was there before with new ways of administering them. And, really, there's been no real breakthrough in the last ten, fifteen years in therapy. Maybe one drug was a breakthrough.

"But during the '80s and '90s, we had a whole group of new drugs—maybe eight or ten drugs, even more, came out all at once in a decade. It was very exciting because the treatments were really very dismal prior to that, and people had to deal with only a few drugs, and very few drugs were approved for migraine.

"Things changed in the '90s when we got approval for many of the drugs called triptans. Seymour was quite involved with the triptan research. Earlier, he was involved with this drug called propranolol (Inderal). Seymour did the basic research, and he was responsible for getting the drug approved for migraine.

"It finally got FDA approval, and a lot of patients made substantial progress in their treatment with these drugs. So he was really instrumental in bringing propranolol into the treatment regimen of headache patients.

"Seymour was very helpful to me when I started my own headache clinic—a small clinic in Westchester County, New York. But I didn't do what Seymour did. He did a lot of inpatient work. He had patients with very severe headaches who would stay in the hospital for a period of time. But I didn't want to do that, so I just set up an outpatient clinic.

"Seymour was very helpful and gave me a lot of pointers. And, also, because it was expensive to … open a new clinic, Seymour was able to help me get some clinical trials. He was familiar with the people in the pharmaceutical industry from many different companies. He befriended me by introducing me to them and getting grants for different studies to help when I was building the headache clinic. We were very grateful for that.

"We had a very nice relationship with him because we spoke to him on the phone many times and then also got together at regular meetings for the National Headache Foundation at least two or three times a year for the last fifteen, twenty years.

"We did certainly get to know one another very well. We've been to his home several times, and he was in our home once. There was a meeting in New York City at the Waldorf Astoria, and we took Seymour and Elaine to our home and had a very enjoyable evening with them."

The Elkinds and the Diamonds traveled extensively, following headache meetings around the U.S., Canada, and the world. In Nashville, they attended a night at the Grand Ole Opry, enjoying dinner with a country music background. In Amsterdam, the Elkinds introduced the Diamonds to the Old Masters through friends who were art dealers in The Hague. They shared pleasant dinners and fine wine in Toronto, Montreal, Seattle, and Vancouver. And in London, they attended the British Migraine Trust meeting where Princess Margaret was in attendance.

Dr. Elkind shares his recollection of a royal oddity: "She had a cigarette, but a very long cigarette, and she had a butler who just followed her all around this meeting. Of course, it was mostly all physicians, so nobody was smoking except her. A butler was following all around while she was shaking the ashes off her cigarette into an ashtray he carried. The butler was assigned just to catch her ashes!"

"Seymour is amazing, and he's still very active," Dr. Elkind concludes. "Very active, and he's still right up there with all the treatments for headache. And even though he retired, he's very active in the National Headache Foundation, the administration, organization, and supporting them as a functioning organization. He's been very instrumental in recruiting people who have become great financial supporters of the organization. Very substantial amounts of money have been brought in.

"Seymour befriended people and helped them with their headaches, and they were forever grateful to him. Many of them are on our board—they're lay members of the National Headache Foundation Board.

"I think Seymour is very much admired," Dr. Elkind adds at the end of his interview. "He has a very strong personality. He's very soft-spoken, but very persuasive and extremely good at management. I think if he hadn't gone into medicine, he could have been the head of a major corporation."

Dr. Elkind currently serves as president of the National Headache Foundation's Board of Directors.

James Staulcup

"In 1978, I started getting headaches," Jim Staulcup, a corporate lawyer, now retired, begins, "and my family doctor sent me to an allergist, who found out I was allergic to every substance known to man. I was miserable. There were points, at times, when I wished I were dead. The pain was excruciating. I didn't know what it was, and I didn't know how to stop it.

"My family doctor finally said, 'You have two choices, either Mayo Clinic or Diamond Headache Clinic.' So, I set up an appointment, and I think I might have boggled Seymour's mind because I came in with a very complete journal on my history of headaches. I guess I'm a little anal-retentive at times …

"My first experience with him was that he told me—and I think I can quote him exactly—'I can't cure you, but I think I can help you.'

"After several appointments we got to talking about various things, and he talked about when the medication wasn't working, there was a procedure that he used for cluster headache patients, going into their unit at the hospital and going through what they called histamine desensitization. And he said I was a classic cluster headache patient. I fit all the characteristics, which I noted by reading one of his books where he describes clusters, and it seemed to be head on. And so I went in and had the histamine desensitization.

"At the time, that meant eleven days of being treated with two intravenous bags a day—I think it might have been twenty-one bags total of solution—where they attempted to infuse histamines in your body, noting that when you were in a cluster cycle, you had an increase in your histamine level, and they thought this might not totally immunize you but would have a similar effect. As it turned out, it did. I went about three years, maybe, that first time, three years without a headache.

"That was a relief, and knowing what caused it also was a relief, that it wasn't a tumor. They put you through the MRIs and all that good stuff just to make sure.

"At one point, after one hospitalization I learned how to do an injection. If I caught the headache coming on, I could give myself the injection and that seemed to abort it. That was one of the things I learned that I could do. Another thing was I could utilize oxygen, and at the onset, I could abort one of the headaches."

The original utilization of oxygen to abort cluster headaches was done by Dr. Walter Alvarez of Mayo Clinic fame, but was discarded for many years until the 1970s, when it was revived as an active treatment for acute cluster attacks.

"Those were great things. Due to his earlier statement to me that he couldn't cure me, I recognized they would come back. I guess at some point they might disappear. I've had probably five, maybe six hospitalizations, and I would enjoy three to five years without a headache. Five was the longest. Three was the shortest period of time that I'd go without one, which was a phenomenal relief to me.

"Fortunately, when the headaches came on, my boss was very understanding. In terms of work, I had to travel quite a bit. I had responsibilities for a subsidiary of AT&T that had units coast to coast. I would have to visit those locations regularly and go quite frequently to one of their big manufacturing locations in Little Rock, Arkansas. I spent many a day down there, had the longest bench trial that went over a period of about two years, 129 actual days of trial, only to have the judge fall asleep each time thinking it was a race discrimination case. And it was not. It was a gender discrimination case. So the other side and I got together, and we worked out a settlement. We figured no one was going to win with this judge. No matter how he ruled, there would be reversible error. No one wanted to go through another 129 days of trial. So we worked out a settlement.

"But I was always antsy about travel because I didn't travel with oxygen, although I could travel with the injections, and that was fine. That improved my quality of life substantially because when you have one of these things, clusters, it feels like someone's driving a hot spike through your eye while at the same time hitting you on the side of the head.

"One interesting thing, as I was returning from National Headache Foundation's board meeting in Palm Springs one year, and while I'm on the flight, returning to Chicago, I started to get a headache. So I buzzed for the flight attendant and asked her if I could get some oxygen. She asked, 'Why?' And I said, 'I have a cluster headache, and it aborts it.' And she said, 'Oh, my brother-in-law (or brother, I can't remember which) has clusters.' So she immediately set up the oxygen. Everyone's looking, thinking I'm having a heart attack, but it abated my headache.

"This was at a time when there were the phones in the plane. You could use your credit card and call out. So I called Merle, Seymour's daughter, who also works at the Diamond Headache Clinic. And I said, 'Merle, I've just gone through a cluster episode. I'm going to land in Chicago later today, and I'm going to come in the next day. Get me in the hospital right away, and get me through the treatments because I know that works.

"Well, I got a call from Seymour while I'm in the hospital. He was very offended that I hadn't called him directly. He said, 'I'm your doctor!' I said, 'Yeah, but Merle's your daughter. You're in California, and she's in Chicago where I am. 'Well, I'm still your doctor,' he replied, 'and I want to know what's happening!' He gets very possessive of his patients. That was one anecdote that stuck with me through the years, *I'm* your doctor!'

"I had good experiences with the clinic. They were all trained in the various procedures for different types of headaches. Some were better at dealing with patients than others, but there was never a question that I could get help there. And I didn't have to go there very often because I had those intervals of three to five years without headaches. It was a great relief. Right now, I keep thinking, because I'm on the edge of about four years without one, and I'm thinking ...

"One of the good things about becoming so closely associated with Seymour was that it seems that when they strike, it's like a Saturday evening and I'm down in South Carolina. That actually happened. We'd just arrived down here, and I knew Seymour was in Hawaii. He couldn't be much farther away than that. I have his cell phone number, so I called up. And his first question was, 'What drugstore is available and what hospital, and give me those numbers.' He called back shortly after and said, 'You're to see Dr. Such-and-such at Beauford Memorial Hospital. Go in the emergency room.' (This was like ten or ten-thirty at night in South Carolina.) 'He knows what to do,' Seymour continued. 'He has a prescription to give you, and he'll call it in to whichever drugstore you want to go to.' So I did that. I got an injection; they gave me some oxygen and the prescriptions to get oxygen and also to get certain medication. So, Seymour could treat me remotely from thousands of miles away.

"We began talking more and more about the National Headache Foundation. I got a call from Seymour one day, and he said, 'How would you like to go to New York?' And I said, 'To do what?' And he said he was appearing on the Ted Koppel show. I think it was *Nightline* or something like that. He asked me to come along as a classic cluster patient and be interviewed.

"Of course, no man wants to go and acknowledge he has headaches, so I gave him some cockeyed excuse why I couldn't do it. It's one of the things I regret the most, not having gone. Something else occurred, and I don't know whether it was when I was in the hospital or how I got to reading it, but I think it was something written by an attorney in the National Headache Foundation newsletter. I chided Seymour about it. I said, here you have a patient that's a labor employment law specialist and knows all about Americans with Disabilities and those acts. So, why don't you use me to write an article?

"That kind of started it off, and then he said something to the effect, well, what about for the clinic? You'd do the labor and employment law. And I said, sure, I could do that. I could do both. I could serve as a lawyer for the clinic, primarily doing labor and employment law work, because I think Marv Cohn at the time was doing general legal work for the clinic, as well as the National Headache Foundation. And I offered to do the legal, the labor and employment law work for them at the clinic, and to write an article for the newsletter. I wrote an article about either [the] Family [and] Medical Leave Act, or the ADA, or the comparable state acts that covered headache.

"That was the beginning of a closer association with Seymour. At some point, I was back in the hospital, and I am a lousy patient. I've got to be doing something. I can't just be sitting there or lying around there all day or attending some of the programs they had. I had to be doing something else.

"One day I asked him to let me see the personnel guide for the clinic. I read it, and I asked, 'Who wrote this for you?' 'Well, we hired a consultant to write it,' he replied. I told him it was a piece-of-something that needed to be reworked. I wasn't charging him for any legal work I was doing for the clinic at the time because I was in-house (employed full-time by a corporation), and I couldn't really do that. But I could treat it as a *pro bono* effort."

As Jim and Seymour spent more time together, they formed a close friendship based on mutual respect and the natural drive each of them exhibits to first notice what needs to be fixed or improved, and then do whatever it takes to remedy the situation.

"One time he invited Karen, my wife, and me to join him and Elaine for dinner at a restaurant called Spruce. It's no longer in Chicago. And I found out at the time that he favored a wine that was called Conundrum that was made by Caymus. I enjoyed the wine so much, but I found out that you could only get it in restaurants or clubs, that they didn't distribute it to liquor stores or wine stores. But then I found out through a friend of mine who had a restaurant that he could order it for me. So, when Seymour opened the headache unit at St. Joseph Hospital, I brought him a case of Caymus Conundrum.

"We'd visit from time to time out of the office," Jim continues, "and he began to involve me more and more, particularly after I retired and Marv Cohn had passed away, to do all of the legal work for the clinic, for the foundation, and for the research and education foundation. And he also, to some extent, involved me in some family-related issues.

"And so he would frequently want to do something with his trust and his wills and the like, but I said, 'That's something I am so far removed from, Seymour, I can't do that for you. But I can get you in touch with a specialist.' So he did, and they've dealt with this individual for probably close to ten years now."

Their close association also meant that Seymour was inclined to discuss personal issues with Jim.

"He'd call me at various times. What are your thoughts on this? What are your thoughts on that? I'd say, 'Seymour, you're the business guy. I'm just an attorney. I don't know how to run a business.' We had some interesting times. I handled some litigation for him, which he had no hopes of prevailing in it, he said, because he thought the other company was defunct. But we ended up recovering every penny because we found out the guy was trying to set something up elsewhere, and he couldn't get a certain license if he had some debts outstanding. So we had a little wedge, and he was happy with that.

"But then he would call me on other things and say, what do you think of this, what do you think of that? And he'd add, 'I don't want your opinion as an attorney.' I'd reply, 'Hey, I have to give you an opinion as an attorney. I can't do it both ways because if I tell you something, it's going to be viewed as legal advice.'"

When Seymour began planning his retirement exit from the practice, he once again looked to his friend Jim Staulcup. (More on that later in the book.)

"I just wish I had his energy!" Jim adds. "He's taken on a bigger task with the National Headache Foundation than what I think he expected to have. There have been two executive directors in less than three years, and one had been there a long time.

"One of the things with Seymour, and it's anecdotal, and I think anyone who's ever been approached by Seymour to raise funds for the foundation or whatever other interests he has will recognize the approach. He'll come and he'll say, 'I'd like you to buy a table for the National Headache Foundation's annual benefit.'

"And you'd say, 'I'll think about it.'

"And the next day you have a letter thanking you for buying a table!

"Oh, he's good, and he's raised a lot of funds in the last two years through various contacts. A lot of people are hesitant and feel uneasy about asking others for funds. Seymour is not. He has a lot of drive.

"One more story: Seymour likes chocolate, and I would always give him a hard time because at the benefits, the dessert was always chocolate. I'd tell him, 'You know I can't eat chocolate!'

"It's one of the triggers I have with the headaches. I haven't had chocolate, real chocolate, since about 1979. I eat the white chocolate because it's not really chocolate, but it tastes like chocolate.

"There's a candy store in Geneva, Illinois, where we have a place with phenomenal chocolates. So I would send a box of chocolates to him, and Elaine would call me. She'd say, 'Don't do this anymore. He sits down and eats the chocolates, and he shouldn't eat so much chocolate!'

"I said, 'Well, the chocolate was for you, Elaine. It wasn't for Seymour.'

"So I don't buy him chocolate anymore. I think he gets one or two pieces a day somewhere, though.

"He's kind of funny, and he maybe wouldn't want this repeated, but I was dealing with what could be a sexual harassment complaint. I called him up, and asked, 'Have you heard about this allegation?'

"He said, 'Yeah, I told them to call you.'

"And then he says, 'You know what upsets me most about this? No one's made a claim like that against me!'

"I said, 'No, Seymour, you don't want that kind of claim!'

"He says, 'Well, at my age, I can't do anything!'

"He has a good sense of humor, and he's forever tried to get me to go to a White Sox game with him. I really don't care for the

White Sox. I don't care for the Cubs. I hate to tell you this, but I was a Yankees fan, and I really don't care for Major League Baseball anymore, not since all the suits took over and the clubs folded in whenever year that was … I told him that I really don't have any interest in watching. It'd be a waste on me, so use your tickets with someone who would enjoy it. I think it's rather boring. I'd rather go and watch golf or college basketball, tennis matches, things like that."

Mr. Staulcup currently serves on the National Headache Foundation's advisory board.

Lee Benton

Mr. Benton is an attorney and a migraine sufferer who found relief at the Diamond Headache Clinic, and he served as treasurer on the National Headache Foundation's Board of Directors.

"I first had a headache that went beyond a pure tension headache in the spring of 1970, when I had moved out from Chicago to the San Francisco area. The migraines didn't become persistent until eight or nine years later. I then proceeded to see a series of neurologists in the Palo Alto area and San Francisco for treatment, but ultimately, their treatments weren't getting me anywhere. And I think the reason was that neither they nor I at that stage—because I didn't know about it—focused on rebound headache and the various things that can cause it, including sumatriptan.

"By 2004, a couple of things happened. The headaches were worse, but I also was able to take some time off to deal with them. And so I knew that I should go to the headache clinic rather than just to a neurologist, even if the neurologist had a specialty in headache treatment. I used the internet for a search, and by far the most impressive website was the Diamond Headache Clinic website, not only in explaining the fact that they have both external and internal patients (the latter are at the ninth floor at St. Joseph's), but there were also, as I recall at the time, a series of white papers done by doctors at the clinic that were posted on the website.

"I'd had enough experience by that time with various supposedly prophylactic drugs which had been prescribed for me that I was sort of familiar with them all, and it was clear to me from looking at the white papers that the doctors at the Diamond Clinic were also extremely familiar with them. So I called them and made an appointment. It took about two months, I think … something like call in April, get an appointment in June. But I ended up with Seymour, which I'm very glad about!

"Things got a lot better once I understood the principle they teach you: a lot of bad headaches really are simply rebound headaches because you've used too much triptan or you've used a painkiller too much, and there's some other things that can do it."

Unfortunately, Mr. Benton had other medical issues that complicated his life in general and his headache treatment in particular, a state called comorbidity.

During the standard entrance interview and examination at the Diamond Headache clinic, a questionnaire response led to a prostate exam, which in turn revealed that Mr. Benton was a victim of prostate cancer.

"I was in kind of a crazy prostate cancer situation," he recalls, "in the sense that my PSA in the fall of 2003 was 2.2. By the time I got back in early July and took the test, about nine months later, it was 6.6! I had a radical prostatectomy that fall for the prostate cancer."

And that wasn't all. Reactive arthritis, also called Reiter's syndrome, develops due to an infection and is considered an autoimmune condition. Symptoms include inflammatory arthritis, most typically in the back or knee, inflammation of the eyes, and sometimes lesions, although not all patients develop all symptoms.

"It's a situation where something like 7 percent of the Caucasian population in the U.S., more men than women, carry a gene variation called HLA-B27. It makes you at risk for reactive arthritis if you happen to get one of the six or so things that can trigger it. There are four food-poisoning bacteria that could be responsible, but ultimately they couldn't pin down which of the four got me.

"A rheumatology professor from Stanford, who was the mentor of my own rheumatologist, said she'd never seen anybody in her career who came in with higher inflammation numbers than I did.

"Before long, a tendon in my right foot snapped in half! It's a tough disease. The chances of getting it are about one in thirty thousand, but it has caused a whole lot of trouble in terms of limiting me as to what I can do. I can get around okay, but it requires monitoring from multiple doctors. They have to damp down your immune system so it won't attack … well, it'll attack the joints and tendons, but not nearly as effectively. But of course, that exposes you to all sorts of little infections, so I constantly have to take care of little fungal infections, some bacterial infections, stuff like that."

The problem in treating a patient with multiple health issues is complex, and Seymour began by placing Mr. Benton into hospital care.

"He started me off with eight to ten days at the inpatient unit at St. Joseph's Hospital, reason being he had to break the rebound cycle from sumatriptan. I think then I was taking Tylenol with codeine for pain, and both of those are rebound-causing things. So I went through the inpatient program. It was more difficult the first time, and I think I've done it three or four times over the last eight years.

"Now I don't take painkillers anymore—well, I take Celebrex for my reactive arthritis pain—but I've discovered that, vis-à-vis, a headache problem and rebound, that ultimately the painkiller doesn't do you that much good, so why risk a rebound effect from that? So I just quit doing anything like that. Seymour prescribed a couple muscle relaxants that have helped if I can feel a migraine developing. Where I get nailed, and fortunately it's not that frequent, is when I wake up with one because then it's too far gone for anything like a muscle relaxant to help.

"After that first eight to ten days at the Diamond Headache Clinic's St. Joseph's inpatient unit, I started coming back to Chicago to see Seymour at three-month intervals. And then gradually that changed to six-month spans. Most of them were typical meet with Seymour, go over everything. Now I meet with Merle to go over everything.

"I can't remember exactly when, maybe it was 2006, that Seymour talked me into coming out and meeting with the board. What's crazy, though, is that Seymour made me chairman of the board operations committee, which includes employee matters and financial matters."

The timing involved Mr. Benton in the recent personnel changes, and as did Mr. Staulcup, he credits Seymour with discovering the problem.

"Seymour caught it, watching the financial statements in early fall. But none of us, even Seymour, at that time realized the situation. It really put a pall over the entire staff, as well as being a financial loss."

When asked if he any further anecdotes or issues to discuss concerning Seymour, he replied that there were two.

"He's been a White Sox fanatic for many years. And the funny thing is, I think he's the first North Side Chicagoan I've known who's been a White Sox rather than a Cubs fanatic. But anyway, a few years ago, he and Elaine were going to a bunch of games. I'm assuming that they might not try to tackle that anymore, but the way he cared and all the souvenirs he put together on it, were a real kick for me.

"The second thing is his historical microscope collection. It's mind-boggling. He took some time when a bunch of other people from the board and I were there. He took a bunch of them out, explained from what era they were, etc., and talked through the development of microscopes over time. I don't know that much about medical instrument collections, but I'd have to guess that he has one of the best historical collections of microscopes outside of any museum.

"It's funny, because he said he got into it because Elaine kept dragging him to antique stores for other reasons, particularly when they traveled abroad. He finally spotted one of these and really got interested in it.

"Seymour's one of the most active eighty-seven-year-olds that I know," Mr. Benton concludes, "and his mind is still clicking with no problems. In our families, my wife's and mine, most mothers made it to that age but were heavily in dementia by then. And Seymour clearly is not!"

Seymour adds, concerning Mr. Benton's multiple disorders, "In dealing with people with comorbidities, I believe that you need a doctor who is not only interested in his or her particular field, but who also can become engrossed in all the morbidities the patient may suffer. That's something I've engrained in the brains of all physicians who worked with me at the Diamond Headache Clinic."

(Editor's Note: Lee Benton, sixty-eight, died on August 24, 2012, in Palo Alto, California due to complications following surgery. In a remembrance on the National Headache Foundation's website, Seymour states, "Lee's loss will be profoundly felt at the Foundation for many years. I treasured Lee as my good friend and advisor. Personally, I will miss him greatly.")

Bruce Burin

Bruce Burin was a patient of Seymour's who underwent what Seymour describes as "a bizarre series of treatments" before finding relief at the Diamond Headache Clinic. Since Seymour's retirement, Burin has been seeing Seymour's daughter, Dr. Merle Diamond, for his treatments.

"I was about twenty-three years old. I was driving down the highway. I was in the backseat of a convertible," Bruce begins to describe his first attack. "The girl I was driving with had a twin sister. We were near Philadelphia, on a major highway, and all of the sudden I had this pain come through my eye. I thought somebody shot me from a nearby high rise! I fell to the floor, and they took me to the emergency room. I was holding my eye the whole time.

"When I got in the emergency room, they asked, 'What's the matter?' My friends said, 'We don't know! He's crying. He's screaming! Something's wrong.'

"I got into the doctor's office, and they had me take my hands off my eye, but they didn't know what it was because by the time I got to the emergency room, it went away.

"The nurse suggested that I see my regular doctor.

"Well, it didn't happen again for a couple weeks, but then it started again. I was at home, and they took me to the emergency room. They knocked me out … somebody drove me there and home again. They still didn't know what was wrong with me.

"So at that point, I started seeing doctors. But they all said, 'We've never heard of anybody having that kind of pain and going through that kind of stuff. Maybe it's in your mind. You should see a psychiatrist.'

"So I tried that, and the psychiatrist starts asking me questions like, have I ever seen my mom and dad have sex?

"I said, 'Wait a second. I'm here for a horrific pain in my head.'

"The psychiatrist said, 'Well, you don't know what it could be. It could be something from your past. And something like that …'

"After I got done with him, with one session I realized that that wasn't the route that I needed to go!

"I had what they call episodic attacks, which means you only get them for like four or five weeks in the spring or the fall, and then they go away. In the beginning, I could go into the bathroom and just tough it out—twenty-five minutes or thirty-five minutes—and I could get by with it.

"Next, I saw a chiropractor, and he tried different things on me, but he didn't know what it was, and so the chiropractor— this was about the second or third year with him—directed me to a neurologist.

"When I went in to this neurologist, I started telling him about how I felt. And he continued on, asking questions that sounded like he was familiar with my problem. I said, 'Do you have the same problem as I do?' He laughed and said, 'No, but there is a name for what you have.' He said they call it cluster headache.

"So at that point, he had pills for me, and the pills worked pretty well. I was with him for maybe two or three years when the attacks started coming back worse than before.

"He put me in the hospital for about a week, and they did some testing. He threw his hands up in the air and said, 'Bruce, there's nothing else I can do. I've done all I can for you.'

"At that point, I tried a Chinese healer. They massage you, and they rub all those pins across you. I felt better, but it didn't help my headaches. It helped my emotional state. I tried that for about six months.

"Then I tried natural points healing, where they look in your eye and they have a chart. I was eating all green-type food. You know, because maybe the food that I was eating was causing this problem. I went with that for about a year or so, but it wasn't working.

"Then I ran across Dr. Gallagher, who[m] Dr. Diamond later on hired to work at the Diamond Headache Clinic. I think he trained him, too. So, I went to see him. I told him all the doctors I'd been through and everything, and he said, 'Well, listen, if it ever gets to the point where I can't help you, there's an old guy out in Chicago—he's the best in the world—I'll send you there.'

"So I agreed to stay on with him, and I stayed with him for about a year. But after that year, the headaches went from being episodic clusters to chronic clusters. That means they never go away. I get them every day.

"Still, he said that he wanted me to stick with him, and I would keep calling there to the nurses because I was in and out of the emergency rooms all the time. They didn't want to see me there anymore because they thought I was trying to get drugs.

"So, the nurse told me the last time I went in to see Dr. Gallagher, 'Listen, don't go into the patient room. Go into his office and demand that he send you to Chicago.'

"Dr. Gallagher was looking for me in the patient room. He says, 'What are you doing in my office?'

"I said, 'We need to talk.' And he sat. And at that point, I actually physically kicked his desk. And I said, 'Look, you've got to send me out there because you're not doing any good for me now.'

"So he agreed to send me out there.

"But what was funny was, the day that I arrived out there to go to see Seymour, Dr. Gallagher started work there that day!

"And the deal was Seymour told him, 'He's my patient now. You had him for a year. Let me take care of him.'

"I found out when I was out there, after talking with Dr. Diamond, that he had this infusion type of therapy where they put these twenty-one bottles in me by IV. It makes you immune to histamine, and that was where most of the pain was coming from—the histamine part of it.

"He did that and it worked for a little while. The treatment, he told me, could last for six weeks to a couple of years. Well, in the twenty-something years I dealt with them, I had it done sixteen or seventeen times, but that was my last ditch effort. When I couldn't get it under control, I had to go in there. Otherwise, I'd be in and out of the emergency room all the time.

"The whole thing with Dr. Diamond was, I could be in there screaming and crying, and he would come right into that room and tell them nurses, 'You stay with him. Don't leave him in his condition.' The way he treated me was unbelievable. I never had that type of care in my life. And you know, if it weren't for him, I wouldn't be here today.

"They call it a suicide headache. There are a lot of people that try to kill themselves, and I've been in a room with these guys. I've seen 'em try to kill themselves. They'd run their head right into the wall. I would never have made it if I didn't have him.

"Probably in my fifth or sixth year of seeing him, I was still having the headaches and I needed them to stop, so somebody told me about this brain surgery that they were doing. He called me in his office. He made three phone calls. One to a federal judge that had it done and told me, 'Don't get it done. It doesn't work.' And the other two people—I don't remember what their names were—but he did call two other people and they all testified to me, 'Don't get it done.'

"I put that idea on the shelf for about ten years. Well, I wound up with a girl … I wanted to marry. And another woman I know ran across a guy that had the operation done, and he said it worked for him. So I called the guy up, and he said, 'Yeah, it worked. I don't get the headaches anymore.'

This doctor was in Pittsburgh—Dr. Jannetta—and he has a procedure called the Jannetta procedure. I asked Dr. Diamond about it, and he swore to me not to get it done.

"I didn't listen to him. And I got it done."

The Jannetta procedure Bruce describes is also called microvascular decompression, and it's used to treat trigeminal neuralgia. The trigeminal nerve is responsible for sensory information, such as pressure, temperature, and pain in the face above the jawline.

It was originally described by Nicholas Andre in the mid-1700s, and in 1891 a procedure was devised to treat it. In 1925 (the year Seymour was born), Walter Dandy used a similar procedure and, in 1932, introduced the theory that the pain was caused by a blood vessel pressing against a nerve.

Peter Jannetta, using microscope technology not available when Dandy reached his conclusion, confirmed Dandy's findings. He then devised a surgical procedure in which he'd move the blood vessel away from the nerve and place a soft sterile sponge in its place to isolate the nerve from contact with the blood vessel.

In 1996, Dr. Jannetta claimed in *The New England Journal of Medicine* a success rate of more than 80 percent of his subjects receiving complete relief and another 16 percent finding partial relief. A follow-up survey taken ten years later shows that 68 percent found excellent or good relief from the operation.

Unfortunately, Bruce Burin was not one of the success stories.

"It made things worse. For a year, I had to sleep on a recliner, and the headaches got worse. I was back at Dr. Diamond's a couple months after the operation to get his IV treatment done again.

"Right now, I'm fifty-nine," Bruce continues. "He also told me that when I got to be fifty that these things will die down. Some of the other patients said the same thing. Sure enough, when I got to be fifty, I hadn't been back to the hospital for any more treatments. I still take twenty pills a day, but I don't get them as bad I used to; I'm not going to emergency rooms. The way I get them now is like a normal type of headache, pain-wise.

"A lot of the time when new patients would come in, if they were younger, Dr. Diamond would ask me if they could come into the room with me. They were scared, and they didn't know anything about it, and I could help them by talking with them."

When asked if he had any final comments or parting shots, Bruce Burin replied with enthusiasm, "I think somebody should nominate him for Man of the Year!"

Concerning Burin's case, Seymour adds, "Cluster headache is an enigma to the average physician. It affects mainly males, and I described it many times as a disease that men primarily have because God wanted to repay them for giving migraine primarily to women. As opposed to migraine, cluster headaches occur in groups, usually maybe five to fifteen headaches a day, usually localized under one eye (not both), and they produce a severe, unbearable pain that may occur continually for two or three months. There is a rarer condition known as chronic cluster headache, where the attacks are persistent and the patient, in many cases, becomes suicidal. Chronic clusters are very difficult to treat and need the care of a specialized headache clinic and hospital unit." Due to Seymour's influence, the Diamond Clinic is one of those places.

Without doubt, Dr. Seymour Diamond provided the knowledge and inspiration for many other doctors to begin or continue their study and practice of headache medicine. A number of them worked with him at the Diamond Headache Clinic and continue to apply his methods, pharmaceuticals, and philosophy wherever they practice today.

An even greater number have benefited from Seymour's books (his byline appears on seventy-three of them) and his medical articles printed in other publications, some with other physicians (489, to be exact).

Considering the number of physicians he communicated with directly and the number who passed along the information through their own talks and publications, Seymour has made a huge positive impact on the world of headache treatment.

19. Research and the FDA

Although the National Headache Foundation's mission supports research, Seymour and his Diamond Headache Clinic performed studies of their own.

"Besides establishing the first private headache clinic and having it [be] a multidisciplinary type clinic, I think the important thing is my recognition of various syndromes, their treatment, and how through the years what I've done has been accepted and used by many people," he states.

It began when Merck's detail man Randy Barth approached Seymour and introduced him to Dr. Clyde Strickland, who in turn introduced Seymour to tricyclics, as described in an earlier chapter. Through Strickland, he also learned about NSAIDs (nonsteroidal anti-inflammatory drugs).

"They had perfected the first NSAID," Seymour explains. "Their research department was great in those years. The NSAID was known as indomethacin (Indocin). It's probably the most potent and well-working of all the nonsteroidal drugs and everything that was discovered after. There's nothing else as good. However, because it probably had more gastrointestinal side effects—or possible side effects—it never really took off in the same way that other NSAIDs like Nuprin took off. And it was never a nonprescription drug."

Nuprin is simply ibuprofen, also known today as Advil, Motrin, and other familiar over-the-counter brand names. They are all examples of NSAIDs. Back when it was new, however, the formula was noteworthy, and Seymour became familiar with its use. It would influence his research later in life.

Next, he wondered about allergies and their relationship, if any, to headaches.

"For many years, the medical field attributed headache to allergy. There's many a headache patient who went in twice a week to their doctor for allergy desensitization for their headache. They were treated with anti-allergy drugs, and I always had a personal wonderment about that. I didn't know if it was really true or not.

"In 1976, I undertook a study to really determine whether allergy was a factor. There is a substance in the serum of the blood known as IgE. And we compared—this is an indicator of allergy, the presence of IgE—the IgE levels of patients during migraine attacks, during when they weren't having migraine attacks, and also against a similar population who did not have any headaches whatsoever."

IgE, or immunoglobulin E, was discovered in 1966 by a Japanese couple named Teruko and Kimishige Ishizaka. Its relationship to allergies is explained well for laypeople in a Wikipedia diagram with the following text: "The first time an allergy prone person runs across an allergen such as ragweed[,] he or she makes large amounts of ragweed IgE antibody. These IgE molecules attach themselves to mast cells. The second time the person has a brush with ragweed, the IgE primed mast cells release granules and powerful chemical mediators, such as histamine and cytokines, into the environment. These chemical mediators cause the characteristic symptoms of allergy."

Also from Wikipedia: "Mast cells … although best known for their role in allergy … play an important protective role as well, being intimately involved in wound healing and defense against pathogens."

Seymour says, "We noted that IgE was elevated in only 5.7 percent of the migraine population, which was approximately the incidence that occurred in the normal population. Nobody had ever done that work before. Somebody's confirmed it since that time, but it was my original work. This study cast doubt on any supposed relationship of allergy and migraine. The findings were especially significant because a proportion of migraine patients were receiving prolonged desensitization treatment."

"A cardiologist by the name of Rabkin published on a drug known as propranolol. It's a beta-blocker used for irregular heartbeat and for angina, heart pain. And he mentioned in the *American*

Journal of Cardiology in 1966 that he had a patient that responded to the drug for his angina but also had some relief from his migraines.

Propranolol is a sympatholytic nonselective beta-blocker. Sympatholytics are used to treat hypertension, anxiety, and panic, and propranolol was the first successful beta-blocker developed.

"In about '73 or '74, I had been using it extensively as a migraine preventive, and it was a common practice among headache specialists. I decided that they should have some studies done and that it should be FDA-approved for that use. So, I called the company Ayerst and spoke to the physician who handled the product, Dr. Rudy Widmark.

"I asked him if they were doing any studies on it, and he informed me that two large and famous institutions in the U.S. had studies going for over two years, without any results! They had difficulty enrolling subjects.

"So I asked him if he would like to come out and visit our clinic and see some of our patients who have responded. Probably the reason the other tests hadn't yielded results is that they were 'super' institutions; they weren't headache clinics. They couldn't get enough patients together to do a proper study.

"He spent several days with me in Chicago, and he was impressed and commissioned me to do a study on the case. When he asked me who else I would recommend, I suggested a friend of mine, John Graham, whom we talked about previously.

"We undertook these double-blind studies on it, and we published on it in 1976. We also presented the material before the FDA. The FDA has a medical panel. If they're judging a neurological disease, they have a neurological panel, usually composed of professors of neurology at the various high-caliber university medical schools throughout the U.S.

"I appeared before a panel, presenting the material of eighty-six patients—the majority being mine and a small group of them who were John Graham's—that showed that propranolol was an effective prophylactic for migraine.

"In the questioning period—and you can put this down; I don't care who reads it now—in the type of questions that were asked of me by the panel, I realized that their knowledge of migraine symptoms was bookish and not practical.

"And after they did this, they conferred and approved the drug.

"OK. Now there are two asides to this story.

"One is that today, to get the same approval for a drug would take about five thousand cases, three or four separate studies, and it could not be accomplished without spending hundreds of millions of dollars.

"The second aside is that for research purposes, migraine is classified as classical and nonclassical migraines. Classical is migraine with an aura, or warning. Nonclassical is migraine without aura, or warning. Today, we simply call it migraine with aura or without aura. Since only 20 percent of the patients entered in our small trial were classical migraine patients, one of the panel members suggested that they only approve it for migraine without aura, or nonclassical migraine. The average physician at that time would not be aware of the difference in its use in migraine, classical or nonclassical. I did not object to it although it is my belief to this day that it is all the same disorder.

"I'm of the belief even today, although many of my colleagues would argue with me, that it's all the same disease. I have sufficient reasons why I believe that, one being that I've followed migraine patients for almost fifty or sixty years, and I've seen them go through both manifestations in the same patient. I don't care what you want to call it. That's proof in my eyes that it's the same disorder. There are people who would argue with me on it, but anyway …

"One of the eminent professors said, 'Let's just approve it for classical migraine.' That's migraine with aura.

"I could have argued with him, but I thought for a minute and realized that would be stupid. It would be stupid for one reason. A doctor prescribing it is never going to know the difference unless he or she is a real headache specialist. The others don't know the real difference between classical and nonclassical migraines. So I decided not to argue about it, and it was approved."

That wouldn't be Seymour's last contact with the FDA, either as friend or foe, not by a long shot.

In August of 1973, an article titled "Headache Expert Charges FDA Blocks Valuable New Drugs" appeared in the *Medical Tribune*. They were talking about Seymour.

From the article: "Asserting that the effort to 'ensure safety for all is to deny therapy to any,' Dr. Seymour Diamond declared that only five new prescription drugs were introduced in the United States in 1970, and 'none of the seventy-five pharmaceuticals which were introduced in England between 1966 and 1972 have been approved for use in the United States.'"

The article continues: "'Unwarranted' obligations placed on the FDA by Congress, Dr. Diamond said, have caused years of delay in the introduction of such excellent drugs as metronidazole, levodopa, lithium, and another half-dozen fine products."

The article concludes: "He [Dr. Diamond] added that the exclusion of certain drug uses 'intimidates the headache practitioner and leaves him liable to malpractice lawsuits.'"

"Up until 1975, the only acute drug used to treat the migraine attack—the attack itself—was either an ergot-related drug or a pain-relieving drug. In 1976, Harold Levine, who was a corporate officer and researcher with a now nonexistent company, Cooper Labs, came to me with a combination drug, which he called Midrin. It's a combination of isometheptene (a vasoconstrictor), acetaminophen (Tylenol), and dichloralphenazone (a mild, nonaddictive sedative).

"I did a double-blind crossover study in 1976, which showed the value of this drug in people for whom we didn't want to use an ergotamine because they may be prone to heart or stroke issues. You wouldn't want to use that strong a drug. Propranolol became extensively used by headache specialists over the years. Amatriptyline is probably the most prescribed drug in the world for pain, whether it is chronic migraine or chronic pain. It's generic, and I credit my original work for that. I picked up on it from a Dr. Lance, who made an obscure reference to it in an article in the journal *Headache* in 1964. [*Headache* is a publication of the American Association for the Study of Headache, renamed the American Migraine Association in 2000.] I also talked about it in the *Illinois Medical Journal* in 1963 and in *Current Medical Digest* in 1963."

And here's the surprising part.

"The use of it is not recognized by the FDA," Seymour explains. "This is an off-market use, even though it is the most used drug!

"That's due to the peculiarities of our government rules. Everybody was using the drug mainly because of my original work, and it became more and more used throughout. But it was FDA-approved only as an antidepressant. Not a pain reliever, or use for headache, or use for chronic pain. If anybody wanted to use an advertised drug for a nonlabel use [in this case, other than an antidepressant], they would have to do a new study.

"Despite that, today it is the most-used drug for chronic headache.

"I have approached the FDA. In order to get its approval at this point for the other uses, extensive, expensive studies would have to be done. But nobody wants to do it because it's generic. They don't want to spend the money. Only a new drug brings them money.

"This is a fallacy in the way we recognize treatments. I went on my own to the FDA about five years ago and talked to Russell Katz, the director of neurology products who does the approval on headache and epileptic drugs.

"I discussed the ridiculousness of not recognizing something like amatriptyline, which has been proven in the field, while we'll spend billions of dollars on new drugs that may have questionable effectiveness. A prime example is the SSRI drugs (Prozac). Because of advertising and expensive pharmaceutical detailing of physicians, billions are spent over the years when a simpler drug, such as amatriptyline, would be of help.

"When you have a general physician or somebody that's not totally educated about the specifics of headache treatment, a representative from a pharmaceutical company (for example) comes in and tells them about a drug A or drug B, and how good it is for chronic headache. And the physicians don't know they should try a drug like amatriptyline because there's no way they can advertise it. Millions of dollars are spent on other drugs that aren't as effective. I think the FDA should do more to make physicians aware of this.

"By the way, the FDA established a lectureship, an opportunity to speak before their Headache Committee, and I was invited by Dr. Katz and Dr. Armando Oliva to give the first lecture. I spoke specifically about the evolution of headache drugs. I felt very honored by that.

"In 1972, a researcher, who later became a good friend of mine, by the name of Patrick Humphrey, a scientist at Glaxo, which later became GlaxoSmithKline, initiated a study on a new abortive drug for headache."

The discovery is described in detail in an article by Patrick Humphrey titled "The Discovery of Sumatriptan and a New Drug Class for the Acute Treatment of Migraine." The specifics are probably understood only by trained neurologists, but in a nutshell, the research team based their direction on solid methodology and findings by predecessors such as the work of Harold G. Wolff.

According to Humphrey, "By synthesizing and screening hundreds of analogues of 5-HT (5-hydroxytryptamine, or serotonin, which is thought to be a contributor to feelings of well-being and happiness) ... we ultimately identified GR43175, or sumatriptan, although not without occasional tangential excursions along the research path. Having found the compound that we were seeking, we were still excited by sumatriptan's remarkably selective profile of action, even though it had been predicted. Thus, when injected intravenously, it appeared only to constrict the carotid circulation ... without the other effects produced by 5-HT itself of the egots."

Seymour continues, "In 1984, they synthesized this compound, and in '86 they received a patent. The first scientific report on it was in '87. The first clinical report was released in 1988. That's where it got out into the medical literature. Before that, it was in the pharmacology and other literature. In 1990, they submitted a new drug application to the FDA, and in 1992, they got FDA approval.

"In other words, it took from 1972 to 1992 to develop a drug and get it approved. Twenty years. That's a long time!

"There's been a lot of comment about the high price of drugs. And sumatriptan was really expensive compared to other drugs at that time. But you have to realize (and I think the public should realize because of this history) why research is important. And that's the point I'm trying to make. It takes time to develop a drug, and you don't know how many clinical trials are going to produce useful results, either. Not every drug turns out like this one, a success story.

"Propranolol and sumatriptan were the big things that brought about a revolution in headache treatment," he concludes.

Seymour and the Diamond Headache Clinic performed numerous tests and studies over the years, often breaking new ground in the study of headache treatment.

They provided a study for Merck that smoothed the way for approval of Triavil, a combination of two drugs, amitryptiline (a tricyclic antidepressant) and perphenazine (a conventional antipsychotic). Seymour has treated chronic headache patients successfully with Triavil since he completed his original research.

They also researched postcoital headache treatments and found that the NSAID indomethacin was an effective treatment and published the results of that study in 1971.

Regarding the postcoital or exertion-based headache treatment, Seymour adds, "If this occurs, the patient should have a careful neurological and radiological exam because any type of exertion-based headache (like we talk about in postcoital headache) can have an organic cause, although thankfully it's rare. Not because of the exertion itself. If, for example, there's an aneurysm or something like that in the brain, it can cause an exertion-based headache as well."

They even undertook a potentially controversial study with an African American population in 1972 and determined that there was no difference in headache occurrence or treatment due to race.

"In 1973, I wrote and talked about low spinal fluid pressure headaches. After undergoing a spinal tap for anesthesia purposes, sometimes a slow leak of the spinal fluid occurs. So people—if they did a block for pregnancy and took fluid out or they did some type of anesthesia procedure—would get a low spinal fluid pressure headache. I described the symptoms which had not been described clearly before.

"Basically, when somebody with that type of headache is lying flat, they don't get it, but in changing positions to sitting or standing up, the headache occurs. But nobody had recognized it before then."

Another difficult subject is the effect of food on headache. Seymour and his clinic tackled this one in 1978.

"Let me say this," Seymour begins. "No clinical problem is more perplexing than the relationship with food and beverages to the production of migraine. A great deal of folklore exists on this subject.

"I did some double-blind studies that show that diet was not really effective, but dietary studies are very difficult to do. People don't conform to it. It has to be done under long-term basis and my clinical experience is that. Over all the years I've practiced, a migraine diet is helpful to about 30 percent of the patients."

Seymour's findings are summarized and presented on the website for the National Headache Foundation.

Tyramine, a vasoactive amino acid found in foods, is one of the dietary triggers that has been found to cause headaches. Tyramine occurs naturally in certain foods, but increases when they are aged, fermented, stored for long periods of time, or are not fresh.

Some foods that contain high levels [of] tyramine are:

Red wines and most alcoholic beverages

Aged cheeses and processed meats (including pizza and hot dogs)

Peanuts

Chicken livers

Pickled foods

Sourdough bread

Bread and crackers containing cheese

Broad beans, peas, lentils

Sufferers who believe that tyramine triggers their headaches can try a low-tyramine diet to determine which foods on the list might be causing their headaches.

Food additives, or substances added to food to preserve flavor or enhance appearance, can also trigger headaches. Examples of foods that contain additives are:

Processed meats

Foods that contain yellow (annatto) food coloring

Canned or processed foods

Chinese foods

Tenderizer

Soy sauce

"During the early 1970s," Seymour says, introducing a new subject, "I worked on the early clinical research with a new compound, indomethacin, which was the first introduced of a group of pain and inflammatory relievers known as nonsteroidal anti-inflammatory drugs (NSAIDs). Although my initial experience involved indomethacin in the treatment of osteoarthritis, I used it effectively in patients with benign exertional headaches. I presented my findings on the latter at the International Headache Congress in 1980. Exertional headache should always be a warning to both the patient and physician of possible organic causes for the symptoms. Once these morbid causes have been ruled out, indomethacin is considered the drug of choice for these cases. Later in my career, I will report of the efficacy of indomethacin in controlling orgasmic headaches.

"In 1976, a Norwegian doctor, Ottar Sjaastad, published an isolated article on what he called 'paroxysmal hemicrania.' He described a case where women (although the disease has since been reported occurring in men) had a one-sided headache. They suffered short severe jabs lasting from one minute to five minutes, multiple times per day. It never changed sides, no nausea, no vomiting, but the most characteristic clinical finding is the frequency of the attacks. They would get usually sixteen or eighteen attacks every twenty-four hours. And he stated that they are benefited with aspirin-like compounds and indomethacin.

"After reading this report in the literature, I confirmed that we had four such cases in our practice. The disease is rare. I communicated with Dr. Sjaastad, and he had difficulty believing that we actually had four cases, it was that rare.

"He asked if he could come over and see the cases, and I was glad to oblige. I scheduled them to visit, and he confirmed that all of them were chronic paroxysmal hemicrania.

"Dr. Sjaastad could not believe, when he came in to see us, that we saw as many patients and treated them as well as we did and was critical of the way we practiced as compared to the European way of spending two hours with each patient. But he published our results with some of his, and other results in 1980.

"In 1981, I described a cluster headache variant by that name, and we published the article 'Cluster Headache Variant: Spectrum of a New Headache Syndrome' in the *Archives of Neurology*, which is one of the foremost medical journals. We described it being like a cluster headache but at an atypical location. It had multiple jabs occurring only for a second, and it had possibly vascular headache, like migraine, related to it. And we discussed how these not-so-frequent patients were successfully treated with indomethacin with the possible use of tricyclic antidepressants.

"Then, in 1984, Sjaastad and a Dr. Spierings took our findings, published a paper, and called it 'Hemicrania Continua.' I believe they appropriated the disease from us and gave it a new name."

Obviously, losing credit for a medical discovery didn't please Seymour, but he did find some satisfaction in Dr. Sjaastad's ultimate professional fate. He had worked with Dr. Sigvald Refsum, the renowned chair of neurology at the University of Oslo, who'd written his Ph.D. thesis on a syndrome that bears his name. As is traditional in that part of the world, when a person of Dr. Refsum's stature retires, his university position is handed down to his subordinate, in this case, Dr. Sjaastad.

Refsum, however, chose not to grant his chair to Sjaastad, and as a result, Sjaastad spent the rest of his career in Trondheim, an arctic-circle locale where, as Seymour says, "the sun hardly ever comes up." Norway's version of Siberia, perhaps. (Factoid: When we looked up Trondheim on a December afternoon, we learned that the slated sunrise time for that day was scheduled for 9:40 a.m. and the sunset at 2:40 p.m., with only five hours between.)

While research can unearth the secrets of medicine, a doctor can also learn from experience in the field, and Seymour learned one of his more unpleasant lessons in that fashion.

"In 1981, I had a very disturbing experience. In treating migraine patients, I usually don't see too many terminal patients. And my experience has been, through the years I've had two or three patients who have committed suicide because of their migraine and about four or five cluster headache sufferers who have committed suicide. One was associated with a family problem, not with her headache, and the others were probably due to the fact that they never followed up on the proper treatment.

"I received a call that a young lady had a severe, unbearable headache. She had initially seen me about two weeks prior. She was a young Asian woman from the University of Chicago, a student. She'd been to several other doctors. Finally she was referred to the Diamond Headache Clinic. On her first visit, I ordered a CT scan, which was negative.

"On this Friday morning, I examined her, and she was actually screaming from the severity of the pain. It was awful. I immediately admitted her to my unit at Bethany (the hospital [with] which I was affiliated at the time). She had intractable pain that didn't follow a migraine pattern—she'd never had headaches before—so I ordered a CT scan on her immediately.

"And as they brought her back to her room, she went into a coma! I thought it was drug-induced. I returned to the hospital after office hours, but she never regained consciousness and she died shortly after midnight. The autopsy revealed a tumor near the cerebellum, which had herniated. There was nothing I could have done," Seymour concludes sadly.

"Working in both the pharmacology and neurology departments of Chicago Medical School, I became acquainted with a clinical pharmacologist, A. David Mosnaim, Ph.D. During the 1980s and 1990s, we published numerous articles about the monoamine oxidase inhibitors (MAOIs) [and] enkephalins (the body's naturally occurring opioids which block pain), and their role in migraine and pain."

Seymour continued treating and studying headache disorders, publishing as he learned new information worth sharing with the medical community. His practice was driven by the fact that he believed all patients' symptoms and complaints were real until proven otherwise. Among the discoveries he published were the olfactory aura when migraine patients' early warning (aura) came as an unpleasant odor. In yet another paper, he described "The Hallucinations of Migraine" when patients were warned of their oncoming migraines by a hallucination.

"I was really a fanatic about writing in publications during those years," Seymour recalls, "the late '70s and '80s. I would get up on a Saturday morning at 5:00 a.m. and work until about 1:00 p.m., both Saturday and Sunday."

Conn's Current Therapy is a book that "offers expert guidance on the latest therapeutic options for common and not-so-common health concerns," according to its sales pitch, and "still the book for practicing physicians," according to Seymour. In 1985, Conn's asked Seymour to write the chapter on headache, and of course, he did.

"In '92, I did the original article on transnasal butorphanol. That's the drug that came back to haunt me. People became addicted to it, and it was marketed as a nonaddictive drug!

"I used it for the acute pain treatment of headache. It wasn't an abortive drug; it was a pain drug. And because of my work with it, it became commonly used as a headache pain drug.

"It was supposed to be nonaddicting, but patients became addicted to it. It caused symptoms like euphoria and need for medicine. I found myself seeing patients—not my own, patients from other doctors—who had used it indiscriminately and who needed to be detoxified. And because of the numerous cases where the doctors had not prescribed it correctly, the FDA finally changed the narcotic classification to a higher warning level."

In some instances, Seymour's research coincided with that of the National Headache Foundation.

"In 2001, the National Headache Foundation, with the cooperation of several pharmaceutical companies, set up the American Migraine Study II. We surveyed a large population survey of migraine sufferers, their symptoms, their records, and their treatments. It involved hundreds of thousands of people."

It was an impressive effort indeed, and it took the pulse of migraine in America. Here's an abstract on the study as seen on the National Institutes of Health website (nih.gov):

Migraine diagnosis and treatment: results from the American Migraine Study II."—Lipton R.B., Diamond S., Reed M., Diamond M.L., Stewart W.F.

Department of Neurology, Albert Einstein College of Medicine, Bronx, NY, USA.

Abstract

OBJECTIVE: A population-based survey was conducted in 1999 to describe the patterns of migraine diagnosis and medication use in a representative sample of the U.S. population and to compare results with a methodologically identical study conducted ten years earlier.

METHODS: A survey mailed to a panel of twenty thousand U.S. households identified 3577 individuals with severe headache meeting a case definition for migraine based on the International Headache Society (IHS) criteria. Those with severe headache answered questions regarding physician diagnosis and use of medications for headache as well as headache-related disability.

RESULTS: A physician diagnosis of migraine was reported by 48% of survey participants who met IHS criteria for migraine in 1999, compared with 38% in 1989. A total of 41% of IHS-defined migraineurs used prescription drugs for headaches in 1999, compared with 37% in 1989. The proportion of IHS-defined migraineurs using only over-the-counter medications to treat their headaches was 57% in 1999, compared with 59% in 1989. In 1999, 37% of diagnosed and 21% of undiagnosed migraineurs reported 1 to 2 days of activity restriction per episode (P<.001); 38% of diagnosed and 24% of undiagnosed migraineurs missed at least 1 day of work or school in the previous 3 months (P<.001); 57% of diagnosed and 45% of undiagnosed migraineurs experienced at least a 50% reduction in work/school productivity (P<.001).

CONCLUSIONS: Diagnosis of migraine has increased over the past decade. Nonetheless, approximately half of migraineurs remain undiagnosed, and the increased rates of diagnosis of migraine have been accompanied by only a modest increase in the proportion using prescription medicines. Migraine continues to cause significant disability whether or not there has been a physician diagnosis. Given the availability of effective treatments, public health initiatives to improve patterns of care are warranted.

In 2003, Pulitzer-nominated investigative reporter Barry Meier wrote an article for *The New York Times* called "The Delicate Balance of Pain and Addiction." He also wrote a book that echoed his research on the subject called *Pain Killer—A "Wonder" Drug's Trail of Addiction and Death.* Both criticized the misuse of the drug oxycodone.

First produced in the U.S. in a time-release formula by Purdue Pharma of Stamford, Connecticut, under the brand name OxyContin, oxycodone is an opioid analgesic medication that has been synthesized from the opium-derived drug thebaine. It is effective in managing moderate to severe pain and has been found to improve quality of life for people suffering various types of acute or chronic discomfort. As other pharmaceutical companies hopped on the bandwagon, they created combinations of oxycodone with acetaminophen or NSAIDs. Percodan and Percocet are examples, although there are many more.

Oxycodone was originally synthesized in Germany in 1916 shortly after Bayer had stopped the mass production of heroin when its dangers were discovered. They'd hoped that a thebaine-derived formula would provide the pain-relieving qualities of heroin and morphine without the danger of narcotic dependence. They were somewhat successful, although only in the sense that oxycodone doesn't have the same immediate effect nor does the effect last as long.

Meier contended, however, that the drug was being used and misused in a variety of ways. In recent years, traces of the drug had been detected repeatedly in the autopsies of drug overdose victims. And this occurred while the pharmaceutical companies were understating its addicting effect and offering the advice of experienced doctors as evidence to its safety.

And that's where Seymour entered the picture.

"They took my statement out of context and used it in their advertising to the medical profession. By that time, I had established my name in the headache field, so my opinions were considered credible. At the time, the drug firms hired doctors to go around speaking for them, endorsing their products. The doctors that went around speaking for OxyContin had a presentation slide showing my distorted quote in it.

"I was deposed in Chicago on this item. It was very interesting. The government wanted to interview me. I had a deposition in Chicago prior to anything else happening. You know there are two kinds of depositions: one kind is 'evidence deposition,' and the other one is called 'exploratory.' This was an exploratory deposition.

"Prior to it, the U.S. attorney who was on the case came in to talk to me. The attorney for Purdue Pharma also wanted to talk to me prior to my deposition.

"It's all in Barry Meier's book *Pain Killer*, about the millionaires and the millions of dollars they made on this product.

"I couldn't charge the government for my time, but I charged Purdue Pharma for my time doing an hour interview with their attorney prior to my testimony.

"I've never seen so many lawyers in my life as when I went in for my deposition. And the reason is that not only were they being sued by the federal government, but [by] multiple states because OxyContin had a gigantic addiction problem.

"I testified that I was perturbed about the way I was misquoted and misused, and that it was a defamation of my authenticity as an expert. I was really disturbed that they used my name in that way.

"Then I didn't hear anything more about it. I read in the papers that Purdue Pharma had paid a big federal penalty and promised to make their drug less addicting. But I didn't really follow it until about two years after this article appeared.

"It was about eight-thirty in the morning, and I got a call from the concierge at our apartment building. And he said, 'The federal marshal is here for you.'

"I said, 'I'll come down.' And down I went down, but not before I said, 'Elaine, bail me out.' Jokingly.

"I went down there and the marshal said, 'Sorry, doctor, I have to serve this to you. They want you to testify.'

"There was a trial going on in Virginia, an action against Purdue Pharma, and I had just received a subpoena to testify. I called the federal attorney who had subpoenaed me, and I asked, 'Can't I give the information in a deposition or some other way?'

"But she said to me, 'This is a grand jury testimony.' Before a federal grand jury. I had no choice but to go.

"I was called to speak, and she asked me to give them my name and my address. And then she asked me, 'What's your social security number?'

"And I said 'I'm not going to give it to this group of people!' [Laughs.]

"She says, 'You have to, by law.' So I did. Who knows who these characters are? Supposedly they're upstanding citizens, but who knows that in the future somebody might use it in a bad way?

"I gave the testimony. It was about ten minutes long. And then I flew back to Chicago. It took almost three days to fly down there, deliver my testimony, and then come back."

20. Fame

With the clinic's growing notoriety for headache treatment, Seymour became a celebrated source of information about the new specialty, and he often appeared on television as a guest expert on the subject. "When I first started at the headache clinic and my first layman's book *More Than Two Aspirin* was published, I received a call from the *Today* show. It was very early in my career, and they asked if I would like to be interviewed about headaches. So Elaine and I flew to New York. I took her with me; I didn't think she'd want me to go alone. We flew to New York, and the network paid for our room that night at The Plaza.

"I arrived at the studio early in the morning. They started about 6:00 or 6:30 a.m., and I waited in the green room. The producer came in and said the show was on, and that one of their female personalities was planning to interview me, not a long interview, one of their six-minute segments. I was told she'd like to talk to me before the interview, so they brought me into another room. It had a television screen there so she could watch what's going on with the show while talking with me.

"We did the interview, and they took an advertising break. And she said 'You know, Dr. Diamond, I'm having a little party at my house tonight, and I was wondering if you'd like to come.'

"I said 'Oh, that's wonderful! Do you mind if I bring Mrs. Diamond?'

"'Invitation cancelled!' she said, and left the room. I wasn't sure what to make of that, but I had to wonder ...

"When I went back to my hotel, we had breakfast, and I told Elaine about this episode. We decided to have lunch that day at a restaurant, a French café that was highly recommended to us. We agreed to meet at 1:00 p.m. there. She was going to be doing some shopping, and I had some paperwork to do. I wanted to talk to the office, and I had a lot of things pertaining to my practice to take care of remotely, so I stayed in the room. I went over to the restaurant about ten minutes to one. All the tables were very crowded, so I sat down at the bar and nursed a drink. I was drinking gin and tonic at the time.

"It got to be a quarter after one, and Elaine didn't show up, so I continued nursing my drink. It got to be one-thirty, and I ordered another gin and tonic. Meanwhile, I began talking to the gentleman who was sitting at the bar next to me. He had an English accent and explained he was one of the vice councils of Great Britain, stationed in New York.

"He talked about his job, and I talked about what I did. I just had done the broadcast, and I was bragging to him about it. And it got to be a quarter to two, and I kept turning my head, looking at the entrance.

"It got to be two-fifteen, and he's still drinking at the bar with me. I'm on my third drink, which is not like me, you understand, and this gentleman and I became very sociable. I was fairly young, and he was in his late sixties at the time.

"Finally, he said to me as I turned around for about the fiftieth time, 'Young man, if it's a girlfriend you're waiting for, she's not going to show up. And if it's your wife, it shows a lack of discipline!'

"Isn't that funny? Elaine finally arrived at around two-thirty, and I'd had too many drinks to be annoyed, so we had a nice lunch and wrapped up our trip to New York.

"I went back to Chicago, and I felt very proud about my appearance on the *Today* show. About four weeks later, I received a call from another show called *Not For Women Only*, a talk show … hosted by Phyllis Newman, Benjamin Spock, Aline Saarenen, and Barbara Walters.

"The producer asked if I'd come in to tape the show. Just overnight. Elaine wasn't happy that I was going back to New York alone, but I flew in and did the show. It was a half hour, and it was good

PR for me at the time. Elaine had driven me to the airport, and she picked me up when I returned.

"As I got in the car and sat down … I guess I should never have told her the other story.

"She looked at me and she said 'Well, Seymour, have you decided whether you want to be a doctor? Or a TV star? Or a husband?'

"I replied, 'All three.'"

Elaine would face other contenders for Seymour's attention as they moved forward with their lives, and it speaks well of both that they resolved any doubts about their own lifelong partnership agreement.

Nothing confirms a celebrity's arrival like an interview in *People* magazine. In his first experience with the magazine, Seymour appeared in their August 12, 1974, issue under the headline "The Headache's Big Enemy," part of a larger section called "Medics." This short, two-page article deals with Seymour's exploration into the field of biofeedback as well as his love for the Chicago White Sox. The sign on his office says, according to the story, "This is White Sox Country," and when asked whether he himself ever suffers from headache, forty-nine-year-old Seymour replies, "Only when the Sox lose."

In his second *People* interview, Seymour and his family graced the pages of the March 9, 1981, issue with a family dinner that included Seymour; Elaine; all three daughters (Judi, Merle, and Amy); daughter Judi's husband, Nathan Diamond-Falk; and Seymour's first grandchild, Brian Diamond-Falk. Seymour was fifty-five years old at the time.

The story focused on headache types and treatments, including biofeedback, a groundbreaking method the Diamond Headache Clinic has used successfully in helping patients control their headaches.

Writer Linda Witt explored the innovative field of headache treatment with Seymour, even to the point of asking if the headache master himself suffers from head pain. His response? In Witt's words, "Diamond claims he too gets headaches, but only when his bridge game slumps or when 'nobody appreciates me'—a phrase his staff heard so often they finally asked Elaine to needlepoint it on a wall hanging."

Ms. Witt also asked the inevitable question about hangover headaches. Seymour replied, "You can possibly prevent a hangover by drinking slowly and sticking to Bloody Marys or screwdrivers. The juice in them contains the sugar fructose, which helps burn the alcohol faster. Or eat some honey. My best advice, though, is this: Just don't imbibe so much."

The *People* article also included a sidebar that mentioned historical headache sufferers and some of the treatments used by well-known contemporary figures. Julius Caesar, Charles Darwin, Charles Dickens, and Sigmund Freud were known to suffer from headaches. Author Lewis Carroll was said to have imagined some of the more dramatic scenes from *Alice's Adventures in Wonderland* while under the influence of hallucinatory auras that preceded his headaches. Eva Gabor revealed that to relieve her headaches, "I take off my heavy jewelry. It helps almost immediately." Leonard Nimoy reportedly finds comfort in flying his single-engine airplane ("I feel better as soon as the wheels leave the ground!"), while Mickey Rooney claims, "I don't get headaches. I give them."

Of course, one doesn't spend a lot of time as a favorite of the American media without running into a few problems. People handle misquotes and inaccurate articles in different ways, and Seymour, in at least one incident, decided to fight fire with fire.

When one of his patients asked him during an office visit why Seymour hadn't warned him against eating ice cream, chocolate, tomatoes, or fresh-baked bread, Seymour asked him what he was talking about. The patient told him that Seymour's name had appeared in a supermarket tabloid called the *Sun* with a story titled "Foods That Prevent Migraine." Over the next few days, forty or more patients asked the same type of question, all based on the *Sun* story.

In his own article published in *Medical Economics*, Seymour recounts his experience with the *Sun*: "While the story correctly reported that I advise most of my headache patients to restrict their intake of foods containing tyramine—including red wines and aged cheeses—I don't endorse the controversial research implicating the other foods mentioned as migraine inducers. In addition, nothing was said about foods *preventing* migraines."

"Now I was angry. The article had caused me to spend many hours restoring my credibility with patients and colleagues. In addition I was concerned that thousands of other *Sun* readers might be avoiding nutritious—or at least harmless—foods on 'my' say-so. And I wondered how much damage had been done to the clinic, which depends on referrals."

Seymour wrote to the tabloid explaining that he hadn't been interviewed by their writer and that "several of the dietary theories ascribed to me were not mine." It took the *Sun*'s lawyer three weeks to respond with an explanation that the writer's information had come from "a wire service pickup of a newspaper article that was a reprint from a magazine in which Seymour been quoted." The sources had all credited Seymour correctly, but somewhere in the Sun's "editorial process," other headache specialists' ideas had been attributed to him.

The tabloid offered him his choice of a retraction correcting the error or an interview with one of their writers for a new story. "Fearing the original errors would be compounded if I agreed to be interviewed, my lawyer and I asked that a correction be printed in the same typeface and size, and in the same position in the paper, as the offending article."

"The correction appeared three months after the original story," Seymour states in his *Medical Economics* article. "None of my patients mentioned seeing it, but I feel it was well worth the time and the $850 in legal fees."

Seymour made hundreds of appearances in the media as *the* headache expert as his career progressed and the Diamond Headache Clinic and the National Headache Foundation (originally the National Migraine Foundation) grew to their present-day sizes. The public interest in a headache specialist held the spotlight for decades, but now in his mid-eighties, Seymour has stopped doing live interviews.

"I'm not famous anymore," he concludes with a grin, "but I was in those days!"

21. Malpractice and Lawsuits

Malpractice is commonly defined as follows: Failure of a professional person, as a physician or lawyer, to render proper services through reprehensible ignorance or negligence or through criminal intent, especially when injury or loss follows.

Lawsuits are the means we use to settle important, difficult disputes in the U.S., and they can bring relief to a mistreated patient. But when a doctor who has done no wrong is caught up in a suit that gathers defendants in the same way a huge commercial fishing net gathers sea life, the experience can be life-changing.

Here, in Seymour's words, is the story of his experience with such a case:

"Malpractice is a very frightening thing for any doctor. All doctors make mistakes. I've made some mistakes in my life, but I always resent being sued for something that was not my fault, or when they were just trying to get money.

"I'm going to philosophize a little. The system is that trial lawyers get one third of whatever they recover or more. I can assure you things would be different if people had to pay for their own lawsuits or if there were limits on liabilities.

"States with malpractice protection, where there's some kind of limit of what they can extract in a lawsuit, have more physicians now. For example, Texas has an active malpractice protection. They put caps on the amount one can collect, and there are a lot more doctors in Texas now as a result. Illinois is wide open. I mean, they can sue for anything. They can sue for pain and suffering and everything else. There are no restraints in most states.

"Trial lawyers have a very potent lobbying organization. They contribute immense amounts of money to political groups—they're probably the biggest contributors—to protect their right to sue.

"The most devastating case I had was the Rita Richter case. Rita was a young lawyer, about thirty-five years of age. She worked for Chicago Title & Trust, a title company that protects your home.

"I had seen her originally. She came to me for headache treatment, and we managed her very well on a minimal amount of preventive medicine. She had a long history of migraines in childhood. According to my records, she never exhibited a daily headache problem. On her last visit with me, I did a neurological examination and she had no complaints except her intermittent headaches.

"I had not seen her for about a year when I received a call from one of the neurosurgeons at Northwestern Hospital, who was a cousin of Elaine's. He thought I'd like to know that they were going to operate on Rita for an acoustic neuroma.

"An acoustic neuroma is a benign tumor of the seventh cranial nerve; there are twelve cranial nerves. It can cause dizziness, loss of hearing, and headaches, things like that. She had come in to the emergency room at Northwestern with some dizziness and headache, and they hospitalized her and discovered the tumor.

"The surgery and postsurgical procedures were done, and Elaine's cousin, the neurosurgeon who was assisting on the surgery, called me and said, 'She's in the recovery room and doing fairly poorly, but she asked for you.'

"I wasn't treating her, but I made it my business to go see her and to encourage her about getting well. She was intubated; that's where you have a breathing tube. I held her hand, and I felt she was going to be all right. I figured I'd hear from her when she was out of the hospital, a thank you note or something like that.

"But then apparently they had an anesthesia accident with her, which was connected with their extubating her, removing the breathing tube. I guess she wasn't ready for it. You have to be at a certain period in the treatment to do this, and she suffered a massive stroke. Massive! The poor woman. But I knew nothing of it at the time.

"About six months from the time of the surgery, a man came to my office and said, 'I have a letter for Dr. Diamond, but I have to give it to him personally.'

"Of course, it was a subpoena. They were suing me, the anesthetist, the neurosurgeon, and Northwestern University Hospital. I read the papers, and apparently she was paralyzed in three limbs and still needed a tube to breathe. It was pitiful. I felt very sorry for her, but this was the first I knew about it. The suit charged that I should have detected the tumor a year earlier, and that I was negligent in not discovering it.

"I underwent numerous depositions where they went over my medical records and asked me questions. I had one that lasted six hours. The plaintiff got an expert witness, a neurologist who never really treated headache patients, but he was their professional witness who would say that I should have discovered it a year earlier.

"The tumor itself was indirectly the cause of her condition, but the treatment she received at Northwestern was the direct cause: the surgery and the postsurgery treatment was what gave her all these problems. I want to make this very clear.

"Originally, I was covered for malpractice by an Indiana insurance company, Medical Protective of Fort Wayne. I've been covered by them ever since I started my family practice. Several years prior to the Rita Richter event, there was a malpractice crisis in Illinois. Doctors could not get malpractice insurance because the laws were so pro-claimant. So, the Illinois Medical Society provided its own malpractice insurance and asked all doctors in the state to participate.

"In loyalty to the medical society, I joined their insurance program voluntarily. However, there was a glitch in their getting certification from the state of Illinois. So they had to have another insurance company cover all their members during that time, and they chose Hartford Insurance Company to do it for a six- or eight-month period.

"In the lawsuit against me, they sued me because I had not detected the tumor, but nobody could pinpoint the years this may have occurred. As a result, all three insurance companies were involved. I was covered by three different insurance companies for a total of $6 million. So I was a very attractive target for any lawyer at this point.

"The lawyer representing me for the Illinois Medical Society's insurance company was a very bright young attorney, Barry Bollinger. He was very reassuring, especially after all the time we'd spent on depositions and things like that. I wanted to hear the testimony of the doctor they were using to testify against me, so I had to spend time away from my practice. I went to his deposition, and he had no knowledge of headache or its management.

"Mr. Bollinger said I should get my own attorney to represent me as well. I had a very good friend, Leon Gillin, who did trial law, and I didn't know any other trial lawyers. I had seen some patients that he recommended to me, and I had a good relationship with him.

"By the way, there was another physician who was sued as well. Rita Richter saw me for her headache, but she also had an internist, and they sued him, too. But his insurance company settled for $120,000, so he was off the case. He was not insured by the same organization that held my insurance.

"At the trial, the neurosurgeon was not there, but he was represented by the attorney for his insurance company. When I asked about it, I was told he'd moved to Saudi Arabia.

"Mr. Bollinger called me four days before the trial began and said 'Seymour, your lawyer is not on the ball.' I'd become friendly with Mr. Bollinger, and he said Mr. Gillin should protect me by filing a notice to settle. He said if you do this and they don't settle before the trial, you're off the hook. You're informing them to settle within the limits of the policy. They have to respond, but it should have been done automatically by the lawyer. 'Don't tell anyone I said this to you,' Barry said to me, 'but I'm telling you to do it!'

"I asked a business lawyer, one of my closest friends, Marv Cohn, who's now deceased, to oversee that the settlement papers were done properly. He stimulated my personal lawyer, Gillin, to get it done.

"Then the insurance company and I talked to a committee of doctors, a panel chosen by the Illinois Medical Society to review malpractice cases. They felt that I had done nothing wrong, that my actions were completely defensible, and they wanted to defend the case against me, even though I filed the settlement papers.

"So, we went to trial. The trial itself lasted three and a half months. There was a lot of expert testimony. And one of the things my lawyer insisted on was that I appear in court every day because it was a jury trial, and when you have a jury trial, you want to create a good relationship with the court and jurors.

"During this three-and-a-half month ordeal, I was in court every day from about 9:00 a.m. to 4:00 p.m. I used to get up between 5:30 and 6:00 a.m. to see patients at the office, and then after I finished the trial for the day, I would see more patients to keep my practice going during this time. It was a terrible experience.

"An expert witness for the plaintiff, Dr. Raimondi, was the former head of neurosurgery at Children's Memorial Hospital in Chicago. He had retired, but he was also at one time chief of neurosurgery at both Northwestern and Children's Memorial. His sister had been one of my patients, and during his testimony, which lasted over four days, I met him in the room outside of the trial. And he said, 'Why the hell isn't your attorney asking me what I think about you?'

"I asked Barry Bollinger, and he thought it would cause a mistrial. I don't know why, but he thought it would throw the whole thing to hell if he questioned him.

"I asked Leon Gillin about this doctor, and he sort of shrugged it off as well. I think I would have gotten better advice from a different independent attorney. Counsel for Rita was Leonard Ring, a lawyer who specialized in malpractice and personal injury lawsuits. He was one of the most prominent lawyers in Chicago, maybe in the country, but even he wasn't determined to press my participation in the case.

"In his closing arguments, he spent most of his time, almost four hours, on the malpractice and mistreatment at the hospital. He referred to me only as ... I think I remember his exact words: 'As for Dr. Diamond,' he said, 'I'll leave that up to you, the jury.' He was going after the big money; I don't think he knew I had all that insurance at the time.

"Barry Bollinger was a very nice man. He was very competent. I liked him a lot. In fact, his wife called me the night before the trial began, which was a nice gesture, and said, 'Don't worry. Barry's never lost a case.' Which made me worry ...

"Around the thirteenth or fifteenth day of the trial, the night before, Barry called me at home and told me I was in for a traumatic morning. He warned me that they were bringing Rita into the court-room, and she was wheeled in on a stretcher with all the tubes in.

"They asked her a few questions, which she was unable to answer clearly, very slurry and disoriented in her presentation, to show she was badly hurt. And then he asked her, 'Do you see the doctor who treated you originally in the courtroom?' I was the only doctor defendant present.

"They asked me to stand and come forward, and she said, 'Oh, that's Dr. Diamond.' That was a very traumatic moment in my life. It was as if I had been pointed out as the guilty person. And that's the point I thought this trial was going to go to hell.

"The jury went out. They were out for three days, and I had no advice. Barry Bollinger thought that I should win the case because they didn't prove anything. He did a wonderful job of pointing that out in his closing arguments. He did such a wonderful job that when Mr. Ring presented his closing statement, he mentioned me not as determinately as he mentioned the other defendants. And he didn't try to prove anything. Barry Bollinger did a wonderful job.

"My friend Gillin didn't even show up for the closing arguments. And when the jury went out, I really had a bad feeling because when a jury sees somebody as incapacitated as she was, somebody's got to pay, and they're likely to make everyone pay.

"So, the jury went out, and my friend Marv Cohn—who was not a litigation attorney, but he was there as my friend during the closing arguments—when the jury sent to deliberate, he said, 'Come on back to the office.'

"It was about noon or one o'clock in the afternoon, and he said 'Let's talk about it, Seymour.' I expressed my bad feelings about how worried I was. I was really shaken. He said, 'Let me call in one of my litigators.' Gillin was out of it, and I needed advice.

"So one of the litigators from his office came in to talk with us; I don't remember who it was. Marv gave him a short resume of the case, and he asked me a few questions. Then he said, 'Send a note to all your insurance companies that you want to settle it at this point. Within the policy limits.'

"I also called Illinois Medical and talked to the chief officer and had a conference call with their committee. I said, 'I don't think

I'm guilty, but I want it settled because I have a bad feeling about the outcome.'

"Marv Cohn's office, not Mr. Gillin's, drew up papers that we served on the insurance company that afternoon, stating that they should settle the case within the limits of the policy.

"That was a lifesaver for me. The jury was out about four days, maybe three and a half days. About five o'clock in the afternoon, or maybe a little later in the evening, they came in with a verdict of guilty for all parties involved.

"I'd never been more shaken in my entire life, except for one other instance. The day after my prostate surgery, I was informed by my surgeon that I had a malignant tumor and that I should get my life in order. Nothing before or anything since can compare.

"That was nineteen years ago, and I'm fortunate to be here today. By the way, Mr. Ring, her attorney, wasn't as lucky. He suffered a massive coronary artery attack about five years after the trial. And where did the ambulance take him for treatment? To the Northwestern Hospital Emergency Room. At that time, they were doing coronary artery catheterization and experimentally using a medicine called streptokinase to dissolve artery clots. Enzymes are injected into the acute coronary to dissolve it, and it can be a lifesaving procedure. I've often wondered, though, knowing who they had in the emergency room, how heroic they would want to be. Not because of the judgment, but because of the possibility of a new lawsuit. Why would they use something that's experimental, the enzymes, and take a chance?"

During the trial, one criticism leveled against Seymour involved the diagnostic procedure he used with Richter. Her counsel argued that if Seymour had done a CT scan on her during her treatment, he would have discovered the tumor; thus, it was a failure on his part when he didn't. She had come to the clinic in 1976, however, before CT scanning was readily available.

And as Seymour admits, after being found negligent for reasons beyond his control, "I was gun shy." As a result, he invested in his own portable CT machine and had it installed in a large trailer adjoined to his medical building.

"With headache," he says, "if somebody's not getting a daily headache, if there are no neurological symptoms, if their headache isn't increased by exertion, and if it's a normal pattern, you wouldn't typically go into further testing because it's a waste of time and money.

"But it made me make compromises. I thought I was a very good diagnostician. I knew I was able to differentiate [between] what was organic or what was something that had to be looked into further and what can be treated routinely. As far as Rita Richter is concerned, she did not have daily headaches anytime that I saw her. She did not have exertion or anything else causing her headaches. And yet, one of the criticisms during the trial was that I never did a CT scan on her."

The Rita Richter case was certainly Seymour's most terrifying brush with malpractice lawsuits, although it wasn't the only one. There were several less worrisome ones that still required the attention of both Seymour and his insurance company.

"I saw an advertising executive who[m] I treated for cluster headaches. Cluster headaches are known to have remissions. This patient had regular attacks in the spring and the fall, which happens in cluster headaches.

"Then I didn't seem him for several years. Cluster sufferers will only come to you when they're having trouble. Some of them disappear for ten or twelve years, and then they come back. Some of them I haven't seen for twenty years and they come back. And that's the way it works.

"All of a sudden I was served with a suit. The ad executive had seen a chiropractor or naturopath, who said one of his legs is a half inch shorter than the other one. They put a lift in, and his headaches disappeared.

"The suit claimed that I had mistreated him. I was sued, and it took nine years to get the thing out of the courts. It was thrown out. It never went to trial, and I never settled. Thank God for Illinois Medical. I'm not the happiest person with them because of their handling of the Rita Richter case, but they take everything to trial. That discourages the frivolous lawsuits. If they think you're wrong, they'll settle it.

"Next one: I was seeing a young man about nineteen years old. He had seen many, many physicians before he came to me. I took his history, and he had a daily headache problem. He had been on many, many medications, and there had been adequate efforts to treat him, but he was no better. He had what we call 'chronic daily headache.'

"Because he already had an adequate trial on tricyclics, which would have been my first choice, I decided to start him on an MAO inhibitor called Nardil.

"I gave him the warnings on it. He was in his first year of college, and he had a twin brother who was not going to college but worked as a house painter with his father's business. I prescribed this medicine, and my record also shows that, after talking with him in great detail, I thought he should seek psychiatric care as well.

"In my conversations, he was a little distorted in what he was talking about, in his feelings toward people. I probably shouldn't have put him on the MAO, but I always think I can help somebody. He said he was doing fairly well in college, and he took one MAO pill. *Only one.*

"In the lawsuit, he claimed that it totally ruined him at that point. He became the dumb twin. This is a true story! He became the dumb twin and could only do the painting and couldn't study. The pill, he said, was to blame. Since he took that pill, he couldn't study and he had to go to work for his father. And the other, previously dumb twin became the intelligent twin and went to college.

"I did a long deposition on the first time it was filed, and the court threw it out. Another lawyer took the case. And I did another deposition. Another throw-out. And then, a third time.

"On the third time, it went to trial. The smart twin took the stand, the dumb twin took the stand, and they gave their testimony. The jury went out, and they came back ten minutes later. They threw out the case. They made a judgment for me, but you know how much time that took of my life? The insurance company paid me, but I took care of the cost.

"As I walked out, I heard his lawyer say to him, 'Don't forget you have to pay me.' He probably paid to have the third lawyer represent him.

"In the next instance, I was taking care of this lovely teacher in her late twenties. She had intermittent migraines. I helped her immensely.

"Then I received a telephone call, and the nurse who took the call said the teacher was on the phone, crying, and asked if I'd take the call. And I said, "Of course, I will!' In those days, there was a six-month wait to see me as a new patient. Of course, we would take cluster headaches or something acute like a brain tumor sooner, but basically, the average case had a six-month wait.

"I talked to her, and she told me she had a relationship with another teacher at her school. He had back surgery, and since the back surgery, he had unbearable headaches. She was crying and asked if she could get him in to see me. I told her I would see him that afternoon after I finished all my patients.

"I saw the man. I examined him and made a diagnosis. He did not have his headaches when he was lying flat, but it would occur immediately if he changed positions or tried to sit or stand up. This is typical of a spinal fluid leak headache. To help his headaches, the leak needed to be stopped. The appropriate treatment is an epidural blood patch. I recommended that he return to the surgeon who had performed the back surgery and discuss the blood patch. I do not perform these procedures in which a person's own blood is injected into the area of the hole from which the spinal fluid is leaking. The blood's own clotting factors should form clots at the holes.

"I soon learned that no good deed goes unpunished.

"So, maybe eight months later, I received a call from her. She said, 'You're going to get served with a subpoena because my friend is suing the doctors who took care of him. I don't want you to get offended. I still want to come to see you.'

"He sued the surgeons ... he sued everybody over at the hospital. So I asked her, 'Why is he naming me in this suit?' And she said to me, 'Well, he's going to these lawyers, and they insisted that anybody that ever was connected to a case was sued.'

"That's the trouble with our court system in Illinois. Not only was I sued, the pharmacies were sued ... there must have been at least fifteen or twenty defendants.

"Next, I went to the deposition. Usually at a deposition, there's your lawyer or somebody else's and the client that's suing you and his lawyer, and maybe another lawyer or so. You know, usually there are four, five, or six people. I went into this room with twenty-five different people!

"These lawyers collect their money by making it inconvenient enough for people that they'll offer settlements. Maybe they'll get a big settlement in the original case, but they'll make it uncomfortable. They had sued pharmacies; they had sued multiple doctors.

"I went in for the deposition, and they spent four hours on my curriculum vitae. Then they reserved the right to call me back. I spent a total of sixteen hours in deposition. It took a year and a quarter for them to get it thrown out of the court. So you know what a ridiculous world this is. I don't know if they got some judgment, but I was out of it. I had the lawyer for the insurance company handle it for me.

"One last story: Early in my general practice, I took care of a family where the wife was very frugal. She wouldn't want to pay for house calls, and she tried to avoid bringing her children in for an office visit. One time she phoned me and then held the receiver up to her daughter's face and said, 'Cough for Dr. Diamond, so he'll know what kind of cold you have.'

"One day, she was in my outer office and she tripped, breaking her wrist. It was a simple fracture that didn't need to be set, and I diligently cast it and followed up with her on treatments for it.

"Later she called me again. She said she'd seen a lawyer about the fall and broken wrist, and they were planning to sue me. She said that since my insurance would take care of everything, she'd like me to continue taking care of her and her family. And I, being naïve and understanding, did that for her.

"And now I'm through with the legal profession. I hope."

22. Globe-Trotting

The combination of Seymour's curiosity about new ways to treat headache and his notoriety as a headache specialist led Seymour and Elaine into the world of international events.

Seymour's first international lecture was held in Paris, where he spoke before the Internationaler Kongresse Fur Hypnose und Psychosomatische Medizin at Hotel Lotti. The date was April 28–30, 1965.

On their way to Paris, Seymour and Elaine stopped over for a night in London and decided to go to the theater. There they met another American couple who had just come from Paris. The couple described their Paris visit with displeasure, saying that their hotel had mixed up their reservations and had to put them in a different room for the night. The substitute room was noisy, and the woman described it as "something I would never want to sleep in."

Which hotel was that, the Diamonds wondered? Hotel Lotti, they were told, the same establishment where they held their own reservations!

Seymour and Elaine ignored their new acquaintances' comments as those of "ugly Americans" and continued on their trip to Paris, still expecting all to go well. Unfortunately, it did not, and the Diamonds experienced the exact same inconveniences, despite their "nice American" demeanor.

"I have some wonderful memories from some of the trips that we made. I did extensive lecturing back then. One of them was a World Federation of Neurology Congress held in Kyoto, Japan, in 1982. We took this tour with friends of ours, Dr. Robert Kunkel and his wife, Brenda.

"Also in attendance were F. Clifford Rose and his wife, Angela. Dr. Rose was a prominent neurologist and an historian of central nervous system diseases. He's retired now, but he was the director of the London Neurological Centre, the Academic Unit of Neuroscience, and Charing Cross Hospital. We made many visits to England, where they held biannual meetings of the British Migraine Trust."

The Diamonds, Kunkels, and Roses spent time together in Japan, and the three women in particular found time to explore and discover what Kyoto had to offer.

One day they were wandering and, as Elaine recalls it, "We had gone off the regular beaten path where they would sell things to tourists, and we were talking amongst ourselves.

"Now, Angela has a very pronounced British accent, and Brenda and I have American accents. She's from Cleveland. And we're walking down the street and were saying to each other something to the effect of, 'We're a little off where we thought we'd be. Do you think we can find our way back to the main area?'

"All the houses were right against the street. There were no yards. Everything was very tight. And, suddenly, a little Japanese woman stepped out of one of the homes. And she said, 'Oh, could I ask you to come in for tea? I haven't been able to practice my English since the Americans were here.'

"We looked at each other and wondered if we were about to do something really stupid, but she seemed legitimate. We went in. She gave us three cups of tea, and I guarantee she had no more than three cups to her name. She did not take one.

"She said she had been there and had worked for the Americans when they occupied and loved working for them. In fact, she went to the United States and evidently kept working for whatever agency she worked for. But her elderly mother took ill, so she had to come back. She said she just loved visiting with us. So we talked for a while, visiting with her. Eventually, we left, and she sent us on our way in the right direction."

Elaine's pleasant experiences in Kyoto were all positive, including an overall impression of the Japanese culture.

"The Japanese were very clean. We went to more than one meeting there, and I don't want to run them altogether, but it was a long time ago and I may be doing that. At one of the meetings, we would be on a tour bus or a shuttle bus, and the thing I noticed was, they were always cleaning the windows; they were always cleaning the seats, and they did it with white gloves. They were just intent on that.

"One of the other things I remember from an experience at one of the Japanese hotels—they were very, very honest! We had our luggage in the lobby before going up to our room, and somebody had one of their bags stolen. It made a huge story in the newspapers! People were shamed by it. It caused a huge fuss because that sort of thing simply did not happen in Japan at the time.

"Then we went to the art museum, which I just thought was so special. They had Japanese colorations of artwork resembling Renoirs. They'd be paintings just like the French impressionists, but the colorings would be much more Japanese toned. It's hard to explain, but if you had two of them together, you would see the difference. The same kind of art—evidently the Japanese painters were copying the French impressionists—but it was the Japanese coloration that was different."

In June 1982, Seymour was the featured speaker on a junket called Bavarian Passage, which offered a tour of the health spas of Germany and Switzerland combined with continuing medical education (CME) seminars. The tour was presented by the Texas Medical Association, and in addition to Seymour's own lectures, he had also arranged for local headache experts to present headache treatments that were not yet being used in the United States.

The two-week trip visited Wiesbaden and Baden-Baden, Germany; before moving on to Basel, Switzerland; and finally terminating back in Germany at Munich, giving the doctors a relaxing yet educational break from their daily lives.

Seymour picks up the narration again, this time taking us to the United Kingdom.

"We made many visits to England, where the Roses were involved with the biannual meeting of the British Migraine Trust. We were good friends with them. Typically, we'd stay in Great Britain for a week or two, and they would come over to the United States, and we were very social with them.

"The British Royal Family acted as patrons to various medical and social work organizations, and the patron of the Migraine Trust was Princess Margaret. Elaine and I attended some of their social functions where she participated, and it was our pleasure to meet with her on several occasions. She usually made a grand entrance with bagpipes playing to announce her arrival."

Princess Margaret, Countess of Snowdon, was the daughter of King George VI and Queen Elizabeth. Her older sister is Queen Elizabeth II. Controversy followed Margaret throughout her life. After WWII, she fell in love with an older man, Group Captain Peter Townsend, who was her father's equerry (personal attendant). Margaret's choice was considered inappropriate by many in government, and the Church of England refused to approve the marriage. Thus censured, Margaret left Townsend and accepted a marriage proposal from photographer Antony Armstrong-Jones. They divorced in 1978, which brought on more negative publicity. Margaret's health deteriorated later in life largely due to her smoking habit, which forced a lung operation, followed a few years later by pneumonia and several strokes. She died in 2002.

"One year, as part of the meeting, they ran a benefit at the Saint James Palace. That's one of the smaller palaces in London owned by the Royal Family. We were invited as Dr. and Mrs. Rose's guests to attend and to have a formal introduction afterward at the reception with Princess Margaret and to have dinner.

"I would say there were about two hundred people there, and they had the BBC Symphony Orchestra playing Schubert, which was a nice program. They introduced the orchestra and about halfway through the first movement ... I don't remember which Schubert symphony, I think it was his third or fourth. Not the unfinished. But anyway, halfway through, we heard the bagpipes, and the orchestra stopped. In marched Princess Margaret. Everyone stood and remained standing until she had been seated.

"They finished the first movement and they were half through the second movement of the symphony, when of all the sudden, Princess Margaret stood up and said, 'I've had enough! I want to eat!'

"All these people had come, but the reception lasted for only about fifteen minutes before everybody went in to eat, and the orchestra never did finish that symphony."

Seymour also met British author Charles Percy Snow, a physicist and novelist who also served as parliamentary secretary in the House of Lords. Seymour describes him with a chuckle as a "pompous, obese, lordly figure ... and very gracious," who would play a part in a couple of Seymour's stories.

As an author, Lord Snow is best known for a series of novels that are referred to as the *Strangers and Brothers* series. He married another novelist, Pamela Johnson, in 1950. Snow was also known for a lecture titled "The Two Cultures and the Scientific Revolution," in which he expressed concern about the gulf between scientists and literary intellectuals.

On one of Seymour's early trips to the United Kingdom, Lord Snow arranged for the Diamond family to view a lawmaking session in the House of Lords where Snow served as parliamentary secretary. Unlike our congress chambers, the House of Lords is surprisingly small, including about ten individual chairs and three or four private boxes, according to Seymour's description. The Diamonds were led to a private box by a helpful usher.

While certainly a wonderful educational experience, the topic of the moment was the Sexual Offences Act 1967, which discussed homosexual issues. The Diamond daughters' ages ranged from nine to sixteen, and Amy, the youngest, about halfway through the session turned to her dad, and in an uncomfortably loud stage whisper that was heard by everyone in the chamber, asked, "Dad, what is fellatio?"

Their usher responded immediately, hurrying over and issuing a forceful, "Shhh!"

"I looked over at Elaine," Seymour laughs, "and said, 'I think it's time we go!'" And they did, with yet another story to share.

On another occasion, Seymour and Elaine traveled without the girls to attend a meeting concerning headache care.

"We were there at one of the British Migraine Trust's scientific meetings on headache," he recalls, "where they invite different speakers from different countries.

"They were doing a fund-raiser in those years, and we planned to attend, Elaine and I. It was formal. I wore a tux, of course, but Elaine was very undetermined about what she should wear. So, before we went, she shopped very diligently and bought a beautiful gown. We took a taxi to the affair, which was held in the Great Hall of Lloyd's of London.

"And as we entered, there was a man in formal uniform who announced new arrivals, which was nice, and they announced 'Dr. and Mrs. Seymour Diamond.' There was C. P. Snow and his wife in the receiving line. They greeted us, and Mrs. Snow was wearing a sweater, a plain skirt, and a string of beautiful pearls, each one the size of a large marble.

"She didn't really get dressed up for this thing at all, and Elaine said later. 'If you have a magnificent string of pearls, that's enough.'"

As he traveled abroad sharing his knowledge with others, Seymour became recognized as a valuable ally by the organizations that hosted his appearances. In 1981, he became executive officer of the Migraine and Headache Research Group of the World Federation of Neurology.

"This is particularly significant," Seymour says, "because I was a self-taught neurologist and not board certified in neurology. Two eminent neurologists, Dr. Arnold Friedman and Dr. MacDonald Critchley, who were stepping down from their leadership roles, thought enough of my capabilities to appoint me."

Seymour was honored again that year when he was elected president of the Inter-State Post-Graduate Medical Association Assembly. He had spoken frequently to the group, and he says he treasured those opportunities because most of the audience—1,200 to 1,500 guests—were physicians from rural communities, and they were attentive and truly appreciated the opportunity to learn about headache treatment from an established expert.

Prior to the group's election, Seymour had received a phone call from one of the vice presidents of the organization. "He told me I was the first Jewish person to be nominated for the president's office, and he wondered if I would be offended if they said a prayer at the beginning of the meeting. I told them that I wouldn't be at all offended and that I think doctors can use all the prayers they can get!"

In 1980, Seymour was invited to speak at Laurentian University in Sudbury, Ontario, Canada, an installment in the Falconbridge

Lecture Series. Falconbridge Limited is the name of a mining company that has since been absorbed by the Swiss mining company Xstrata. It was originally named after the town of Falconbridge, and the town was named after Judge William Glenholme Falconbridge, son of Irish immigrant John Kennedy Falconbridge. The lecture series was established in 1978 in memory of five employees who died in an airplane crash en route to a company meeting near Barrie, Ontario, Canada on September 7, 1977. Xstrata continues to support the series today.

In his travels, Seymour often occasionally ran into well-known personalities.

"In 1982, I was at the New York Marriott Marquis. It just had been recently built. I was at a research meeting with Arnold Friedman and Frank DeSerio.

"Dr. DeSerio—who was a Ph.D., not an M.D.—worked full-time for Sandoz Pharmaceuticals, which is now known as Novartis. They had a migraine project, and he wanted Dr. Friedman and me to head it. We arrived the night before, and I was supposed to meet them in the hotel restaurant.

"The place was swarming with people because it was a night of a heavyweight championship fight. They had set up a large closed-circuit TV in a private viewing room because they didn't broadcast these events on television for everybody to see and sold seats for it.

"I had no interest in it, but Arnold had expressed to me early in the afternoon that day that he would *love* to have gone, but we had our dinner appointment, and the thing was sold out anyway, so I ignored it.

"Later, I was walking to my room in the hotel, and a door was open to a gigantic suite. I looked in, and a friendly African American man caught me peeking and said, 'Come on in!'

"I went in and saw that he had a large TV screen, and they were bringing up all kinds of food. He had arranged for a closed-circuit presentation of the fight for him and his friends. And he actually had—you know how you set up bleachers for people to sit on? He had a small, maybe four-tier, setup so everybody could watch the fight.

"So, anyway, he introduced himself. He said, 'I'm Lionel Richie.'"

Lionel Richie performed with the Commodores as their lead singer from 1968 through 1982, when he released his self-titled solo album. He'd created several R&B groups during the '60s, settling in with the Commodores in 1968. They garnered an Atlantic Records contract and produced one record before moving on to Motown Records, where they'd stay, gaining more recognition from the songs Richie wrote and sang, such as "Easy," "Three Times a Lady," "Still," and "Sail On." Richie also performed the song "Endless Love" with Diana Ross in 1981, topping the charts both here and abroad, becoming one of Motown's biggest hits ever. Richie, now in his early sixties, still performs regularly.

"I introduced myself, and he asked me about me, why I was there, and we talked, and eventually he said, 'Would you like to come to my suite tonight and be my guest?'

"But I said to him, 'I've got a dinner date with two of my friends. Two doctors.'

"And he says, 'Bring them along!' I knew Arnold would be thrilled.

"So we had dinner with Lionel Richie, watched the fight on his television, and he kept introducing me around to all his friends all night. Afterward he sent me a couple of his albums. And for the next couple of years, I got a number of personal referrals from both California and New York from him. He had his friends call me to come see me. Isn't that nice?

"Another time, we went to Beerse, Belgium, for a meeting held by Janssen Pharmaceutica. Paul Janssen was both an M.D. and an avid researcher, and he now had one of the largest research and product companies in Europe.

"There were about two hundred physicians attending, and I was one of the presenters. At the first coffee break, there was this man who[m] I hadn't met inquiring about me. That was Paul. He came over and said, 'I want to thank you and congratulate you on the work you did on our product in the United States. You were the only one over there that published on it.'

"Janssen is a gigantic company. It was bought out by Ortho Pharmaceuticals in 1961, which is a division of Johnson & Johnson.

I think Paul probably became the richest man in Europe at that time. He said, 'I've got a table with a few of my board members, and I'd like it if you would sit with us at dinner.' They had planned a banquet that night for the meeting attendees.

"While we were at dinner, Elaine and I were talking with him, and I asked how he got into the pharmaceutical business because he was a general practitioner at first. And he told me the story.

"He said he had a number of friends that did professional bicycle road racing. And when they got off their bikes, many of them were hyped up. He didn't know whether it was due to drugs or what, but they were really hyped up and needed something to calm them down.

"So he invented a drug called haloperidol to calm his cycling friends at the end of a race, but the new formula went far beyond simple tranquilization. It was known commercially as Haldol, and it became one of the most used of the antipsychotic drugs. Before its introduction, there was only one other prominent antipsychotic drug, chlorpromizine. It's a strong antipsychotic, but it could be used as a tranquilizer if managed carefully."

And then there was the time they attended the Asian & Oceanic Congress of Neurology in Bali, Indonesia.

"I was asked to speak there, so we went to Bali. At the hotel, we met a businessman who worked for one of the pharmaceutical companies and lived there. He told us we couldn't visit Bali without seeing one of their spiritual services. It was a Friday night, and the show included lots of chanting, walking on a bed of hot coals, walking on a bed of shattered glass, and the renowned dance of Bali, legong, or the dance of the virgins."

According to Bali legend, a prince dreamed of two maidens who danced to traditional gamelan music, and after he awakened, used his princely influence to bring his dream to life.

Legong dancers today begin training at the age of five and perform only before reaching puberty. They are highly regarded, and as adults, they often wed into high society. The dance may tell one of several stories from a collection of heroic romance tales from Bali lore. Seymour's world travel exposed the Diamonds to a broad range of ethnic experiences.

In Seymour's travels, whenever he was invited to a foreign country to speak, except England, there was typically a long lag in having his expenses paid by those who invited him. So, whenever he'd accept such an offer, he always included a letter explaining that he'd like to be paid at the time of the lecture. And surprisingly, that created a couple of unusual situations.

He was giving a talk at the VIII World Congress of Psychiatry in Athens, Greece, and the doctor who'd invited him greeted him right before lecture. After pleasantries were exchanged, his host said, "Follow me." Seymour did. The man led him down the hall to the men's restroom. Seymour followed him in. The man walked to one of the toilet stalls, opened the door, and once again invited Seymour to follow him.

We can only imagine what thoughts were traversing Seymour's mind at that moment, but he did as requested. Once they both were inside the stall, the host unbuckled his belt, opened his trousers, and produced a money belt from which he paid Seymour in cash for his speaking engagement expenses.

Another bizarre experience occurred in Mexico, where the event organizer paid Seymour in U.S. $1 bills. "I felt like a smuggler going home," Seymour said of his travel bag filled with money.

In 1986, Seymour received an invitation to speak at a meeting of the Institute of Neurology, the Academy of Medical Sciences of the USSR in Moscow. The event was sponsored by VAAP, the state's copyright division, in cooperation with International University Press.

He and Elaine flew via Air France into the Russian capital. After passing through customs without their luggage because it had been lost, they were met by a driver who took them to their hotel. They'd been advised to bring a selection of small gifts with them such as leather belts, silk stockings, and cigarettes, which they'd packed in their luggage.

Their luggage wasn't found until the next day, and they were then required to make an hour-and-a-half trip back to the airport to pick it up. Only owners were allowed to retrieve their bags. And when they opened them back at the hotel, they discovered that some of their gifts had already been dispensed, apparently to the state luggage inspectors.

The organizers provided spending money, a daily ration of rubles, to the Diamonds, but they found little to purchase aside from the typical Russian nesting dolls souvenirs.

"When we got ready to leave, we gave our rubles to the guide who showed us around," Seymour admits.

In fact, their view of Russia was largely disappointment due to the lower standard of living.

"There was no traffic on the streets; no one had cars," Seymour recalls. "When our host took us to visit the synagogue, I thought it was a deserted building.

"When they took us on a tour before the talk, everything looked well-worn or obsolete," he adds.

There were three to four hundred people awaiting Seymour's talk, and the venue was packed. "They were standing, sitting on the window sills, everywhere!" Seymour remarks, "I don't know if it was compulsory that they attend or if they really wanted to hear me. Continuing medical education in the U.S. is necessary to renew one's license. My thought is that it was compulsory for all Russian doctors to attend every continuing medical education event."

There was no simultaneous translation of Seymour's speech. Instead he'd utter a sentence of two, and then wait while a translator repeated the words in Russian. He found the slower pace interrupted his rhythm, making the talk more awkward. He'd never had to deliver a talk in this fashion before, but eventually he completed it.

On another day, Seymour was asked by his sponsor if he'd meet with various scientific authors to see if he could recommend which ones would be of interest to publish in the U.S. He spent four hours with twenty-seven "poor souls" who'd written scientific books, reviewing their work and talking with them. They all had expectations that their books would be welcome in America. They sent a shipment of their books, a process that took almost a year, to Seymour in the U.S., and he did what he could to help them.

They were taken to dinner twice by the head of neurosurgery at the institute. He was Jewish, and he talked about Stalin, how he suffered during those days as a Jew.

On the last night, he asked Seymour if he could talk to him. He said he'd been asked to write a manuscript for a neurosurgical paper.

It was primarily American, but he had done some innovative work, so he would do a chapter.

"If I send it by regular channels, it'll take six months to a year to get there," he said. So he asked if Seymour would hand-carry it for him. After the warning they'd received and the close scrutiny they'd been given as Americans, Seymour was worried, but he agreed to do it.

"I could see myself in a gulag," he reminisces. "I had nightmares that night!"

Thus prepared, they went to the airport. Their driver, who Seymour believes was a KGB agent, took them to customs for their departure. Surprisingly, this time the customs agents let them through without checking anything, much to Seymour's relief.

On their flight back to Paris, Seymour recalls overhearing the conversations among a group of French communists. They'd had high expectations when they left France to visit Russia, but their discussions on the trip home expressed disappointment.

Perhaps the most pleasant trip Seymour and Elaine enjoyed together was their journey to Venice to join Bayer AG for a pre-one hundredth anniversary celebration of the discovery of aspirin, which included an unexpected surprise.

Actually, there were two unexpected surprises, although the first, smaller incident wasn't as positive as the one that came later. They'd decided to fly on the Concorde supersonic jet to Paris before continuing on to Venice. Since it was their first Concorde experience, they hadn't heard about the means used by the jet to manage pitch trim for supersonic flight. Fuel is actually pumped from one tank to another, changing the fore/aft center of gravity to assure smooth flight, but when it happens, without warning, the entire airframe shakes. Veteran Concorde fliers don't worry about it, but when Elaine and Seymour first experienced the effect, they thought something was going terribly wrong and were visibly relieved when a flight attendant comforted them with an explanation.

Once in Venice, the Diamonds ran into a personal conflict. The celebration at a palace on the main canal was to be held on the same day as Elaine's birthday.

"You're not going to take me to a drug conference on my birthday," she stated.

"We really should go, but I'll take you out tomorrow night," Seymour proposed. And after some discussion and guilt placement, they attended the Bayer celebration, which turned out to be not so bad after all. . . .

Seymour's Bayer contact, Dr. Dietmar Bahn, after he learned of Elaine's birthday, immediately made plans to celebrate the occasion. He had some help from the fact that it was also time for the Carnival of Venice.

The Carnival traditionally begins forty days before Easter and ends on Shrove Tuesday (also called Fat Tuesday), the day before Ash Wednesday. Originally, it was a time for celebration among the classes, and participants wore masks to erase any distinction between their social statuses. The tradition faded over the years until the 1970s, when the Italian government made an effort to regain the old culture of Venice and positioned the Carnival celebration to be the festival's centerpiece. Elaborate costumes and masks are the order of the day, and an international jury of costume and fashion designers picks a winner, "La maschera piu bella" (Most beautiful mask).

Dr. Bahn did a remarkable job of assuring that the Diamonds had an enjoyable evening. First, he arranged for a water taxi to deliver them to the palace venue, where a team of trumpeters performed a welcome fanfare when Elaine stepped off the boat. In the meantime, he arranged for a beautiful birthday cake to be prepared for her. And then, when she'd entered the palace ballroom, the entire assemblage sang "Happy Birthday" to her. She was surprised and delighted by the attention and called it her best birthday ever.

It was also at this event that Seymour met Sir John Vane, who shared the 1982 Nobel Prize in Physiology or Medicine with Sune K. Bergström and Bengt I. Samuelsson for discovering how aspirin works. The Diamonds and the Vanes became good friends and, as noted earlier in the book, Dr. Vane would come to speak at Seymour's alma mater at Seymour's request.

"I put Sir John up at the Drake Hotel in Chicago and had a special dinner for him at the International Club, a famous private club, part of the hotel.

"Sir John always wore a favorite corduroy jacket. Unfortunately, one of the servers spilled gravy all over the jacket! The next day, he sent it out to be cleaned, and it came back in terrible shape.

"I spoke to the hotel management, and sure enough, they did not argue. They had him send them the bill, and they reimbursed him. In Amsterdam at a similarly famous hotel, we experienced a similar event with Elaine and a dress she sent out. They were not as accommodating as the U.S. hotel.

"In 1998, Elaine and I went to an International Headache meeting in Amsterdam," Seymour begins a new story. "And one of the very memorable things about that trip was they had, as a social event, a candlelight hors d'oeuvre party at the Rembrandt Museum. It was wonderful to see the most famous of Rembrandt paintings, *Night Watch*."

Seymour reads, "The popular legend holds that this ground-breaking painting was unappreciated at its time and ruined Rembrandt. However, he earned a handsome sum from the *Night Watch*. The sixteen soldiers depicted in the middle ground reportedly paid an average of a hundred guilders apiece to be in the picture, and the amount varied in relation to how prominently they were featured.

"Elaine and I took a group of guests—Dr. Elkind, Dr. Kunkel, and their wives—to dinner at one of the finer hotels. Elaine and I at that time were not sophisticates of French food. We looked at the menu, and I ordered routine things, and Elaine noticed they had white truffles. There was no specific pricing; the menu simply said 'market price.'

"They brought a selection of them to the table, all different sizes. Anyway, she picked a pretty big one, and when I got the bill—and that was a lot of money at that time—there was a $350 figure, just for the truffle!"

So, did they at least enjoy the expensive treat?

"I don't know," Seymour laughs. "I don't remember, but I don't think it was worth $350! And that's our truffle story. I remind her of it every time we go to an Italian restaurant where truffles are on the menu."

23. Aspirin

Aspirin is Bayer's name for acetylsalicylic acid. It's a mild analgesic used in the treatment of headache and muscle/joint pain. Postglandins are natural body chemicals that cause blood clotting and sensitize nerve endings to pain. Aspirin blocks the production of postglandins with a two-pronged advantage. The desensitization of nerve endings, of course, eases pain, and the removal of the postglandins' blood-clotting capabilities makes aspirin useful in treating heart patients by thinning their blood.

Early scientists, however, had no idea how it actually worked. That would come much later, when the research of British pharmacologist Sir John Vane and his fellow 1982 Nobel Prize for Medicine winners, Bergström and Samuelsson, demonstrated that aspirin's blocking of postglandin production was the actual mechanism.

Aspirin's primary ingredient, salicin, which is found in the bark and leaves of willow trees, was used by Hippocrates to ease pain. He didn't isolate salicin—it wasn't recognized until 1829 by scientists as a source of pain relief—but even though Hippocrates didn't understand the chemistry, he applied his anecdotal knowledge of the drug to help patients.

Salicin was further refined in the early 1800s, when Italian chemist named Raffaele Piria separated it into two components, one a sugar and the other a component called salicylaldehyde. It was the latter he would convert, using hydrolysis and oxidation, into what we now call salicylic acid.

Salicylic acid, though a competent pain reliever, is too acidic for comfortable digestion in humans, and it wasn't until 1853 that a

French chemist, Charles Frédéric Gerhardt, neutralized its acidity by buffering it with sodium salicylate and acetyl chloride, which produced acetylsalicylic acid, or what we now call aspirin. Although he'd created a useful new medicine, Gerhardt wasn't interested in developing it as a commercial product, and the discovery sat unused for almost another fifty years.

Finally, in 1899, one of Bayer's German chemists, Felix Hoffman, rediscovered the Gerhardt solution and offered it to his father, who suffered from arthritis. Hoffman then encouraged Bayer to produce his new pain reliever, which they named "Aspirin" after the "A" in acetyl acid, the "spir" in spiraea ulmaria (the plant used to produce the salicylic acid), and the "in" was simply a common ending for medicines at the time. On February 27, 1900, Bayer patented their new product.

Interestingly, Hoffman discovered another product that Bayer named "Heroin." He'd been instructed to produce codeine, a constituent of the opium poppy, which is similar to morphine but less potent and less addictive. Unfortunately, the experiment produced an acetylated form of morphine, which was almost two times as potent as morphine.

The name Heroin came from the Greek "Heros" due to its perceived "heroic" effects on a patient, and from 1898 through 1910, Heroin was marketed as a cough suppressor that didn't have the addictive side effects of morphine. Morphine at the time was used as a recreational drug, and Bayer wanted a similar drug without the addictive side effects. They even marketed Heroin as a cure for morphine addiction until they learned that it metabolizes to form morphine. The company was truly surprised and embarrassed when Heroin developed a base of addicted users.

On a less controversial note, Bayer's trademarked Aspirin proved to be a true wonder drug, and it was this drug that they wanted to associate with Seymour Diamond, the world-renowned headache doctor, because of his stature in the headache community. Most medications are replaced by newer, better drugs within a relatively short period, but aspirin would remain a favorite for more than a century.

Bayer, by the way, lost its trademark, leaving aspirin generically named, in the 1919 Treaty of Versailles when the Germans were defeated in World War I.

Seymour had met Dr. Dietmar Bahn when Bahn visited the Diamond Headache Clinic in Chicago. Bahn was a medical doctor, but he worked directly for Bayer AG in Germany, and he came to see Seymour to offer him a proposition.

Bayer had patented the formula for aspirin in the year 1900, and they were planning a huge one hundredth anniversary project to celebrate the discovery. Dr. Bahn asked if Seymour would be interested in writing a monograph for Bayer titled *Migraine Through the Ages*. The project would also include numerous consultations and lectures, all fully sponsored by Bayer.

Seymour accepted the offer and began a period of writing mixed with speaking engagements at various venues around the world, but then a change took place. Bayer decided to cancel the project. They had planned to use the book when they introduced a new pain-relieving drug, but because of the product's toxicity, it was never marketed. So, they signed over the rights to the work to Seymour.

Although Bayer was out of the picture as far as the monograph was concerned, Seymour was inspired by the project, and with his director of administration, Mary Franklin, he completed a book titled *Headache Through the Ages*. That book has become a reference standard for anyone interested in the history of headache and its treatment.

24. Specialized Headache Treatments

Sometimes specialized treatments can be simple. Have you considered, for example, that the morning cup of coffee you drink could also have pain-relieving qualities? It's true.

In an abstract presented at the Ninety-eighth Annual Meeting of the American Society for Clinical Pharmacology and Therapeutics in 1997, Doctors Seymour Diamond and Fred Freitag of the Diamond Headache Clinic, with T.K Balm and D.A. Berry of Procter & Gamble, shared the results of a clinical trial involving caffeine, ibuprofen, and a placebo in treating tension headaches.

In a randomized, double-blind, multicenter parallel trial, 385 subjects with a history of tension headaches, typically three to seven per month, were treated with a combination of ibuprofen and caffeine, ibuprofen alone, caffeine alone, or the placebo.

The results revealed that the ibuprofen-caffeine combination provided significantly better pain relief than any of the treatments alone, and the combination also delivered the relief notably faster than ibuprofen alone.

"Significantly, I showed in this study that caffeine alone gave almost as good relief for the first hour of treatment as the pain reliever or the combination drugs. This established the fact that caffeine had some general effects in many headaches. It also established me as a caffeine expert."

But not all headaches can be treated so simply. In Seymour's book *Hope for Your Headache Problem—More Than Two Aspirin*, he dedicated a chapter called "Man's Most Terrible Pain" to the description and treatment of cluster headaches.

"A typical cluster headache produces a severe, one-sided pain, usually located over or near the eye, lasting an hour to two hours," he says. "Cluster headaches can occur from two to four times a day up to six to ten times a day, hence the term 'cluster.'

"It's the only headache that will wake a patient from a sound sleep, and it brings a sharp, piercing pain, almost unbearable, that usually lasts anywhere from ten minutes to two hours. It's accompanied by tearing of the eye, flushing of the face, and congestion in the nose, all on the same side as the headache.

"Cluster headache occurs usually in the spring or in the fall, although it has nothing to do with allergies and can occur anytime in the year. It lasts anywhere from one week to two months or two and a half months.

"And then there's a complete remission!"

Normally, the remission lasts only until the next year when the headaches return, but it could be longer in some cases.

"I've seen people go on remission for as long as eight or nine years, but then it comes back. That's why a lot of charlatans with bizarre treatments will say they helped these cases or cured them because of the natural remission that occurs."

Dr. John Graham of the Faulkner Research Clinic in Boston, a renowned expert on the subject as a result of his extensive research, has determined that of cluster headache sufferers, 32 percent cry when the headache strikes, 37 percent yell out loud, 16 percent bang their heads on the wall, and another 14 percent fall to the floor, writhing in pain.

"It is this kind of pain," Seymour mentions in his book, "we believe, that led ancient man to have holes cut into his skull (called 'trepanning') to let the evil spirits out. Modern man seeks to escape the pain in less savage ways: one cluster victim will stick his head in an oven, another in a refrigerator, still another in a bucket of ice. And there is always the danger that the pain will drive its victims to suicidal extremes. As one cluster victim told me, 'My wife took the shotgun out of our house because she was afraid I might use it.' Some people call it the 'suicide headache.'"

Each case has its own individual characteristics. Here, Seymour describes his treatment of patient Bruce Burin, who suffered from an unusual case of cluster headache.

"He was experiencing what we call a chronic cluster. Usually, clusters aren't chronic; only about 10 to 15 percent become chronic, but they are difficult to treat, and the patient can become suicidal.

"In Bruce's case, he went all over for treatment before he came to me, and we helped him with our treatments. Bruce's case is interesting because there is a famous neurosurgeon who does a very complicated, high-risk operation for a neurological disorder, not related to cluster headache, known as tic douloureux, or facial neuralgia. Somebody in French literature first described it. It's a type of face pain that is different than cluster. That's what the operation is famous for, but the surgeon has attained a great deal of notoriety for curing cluster headaches by doing this operation.

"However, as I told you, clusters have natural remissions, so I'm always dubious. I don't think I ever cured a cluster headache, and I don't think anybody's really cured it from its natural course. But you can control it and help somebody with it. In Bruce's case, he was sent to a doctor for a cure, but it had no effect, and a costly, dangerous operation was performed on him.

"In my practice, I will use the ergotomines or the triptan drugs to treat the acute cases. Also, I adopted the treatments that were talked about in the '40s and '50s for the acute pain. Bayard Horton and Walter Alvarez of the Mayo Clinic wrote about giving a patient an oxygen tank and having them breathe high levels of oxygen during the attack to lessen or relieve the pain. This technique was more or less discarded by most of the routine doctors treating headaches because they never held Horton and Alvarez in high esteem, as far as headache was concerned. Both of them were acquaintances of mine, and Alvarez was a friend. So we did adopt it in treating clusters. Later on, headache specialist Dr. Lee Kudrow wrote about the use of it.

"Also, in treating the acute attacks, there are patients that are unresponsive to almost anything we can do. These are severely suffering people; you can't imagine. In selective patients, we've used cocaine nose drops, which acted anesthetically to relieve the pain. I want to emphasize that I've used it *selectively*. Most doctors won't. I've never had a patient addicted to it all the years I've used it because of my selectivity.

"At the Mayo Clinic, Bayard Horton, a famous internist, used a form of intravenous histamine desensitization to treat cluster headaches during attacks to break up the attacks. If a person was in a series of attacks, they started this histamine desensitization during that period. Several of the residents, younger doctors who were trained there, used it after they left the clinic.

"One of them was a friend of mine, Robert Ryan, Sr. However, the main headache establishment never really accepted or even tried that form of therapy. And because I wanted to be part of the main group, I had been clouded against it by my older peers, Arnold Friedman and John Graham. I never tried it until I saw a couple of patients who had been treated by Robert Ryan, chronic patients. I wouldn't use histamine for the acute patients. I saw several chronic patients that were dramatically helped by Ryan with this histamine treatment, so I flew down to talk to him and to learn his technique. He taught it to me, and we've used it successfully at the Diamond Headache Clinic for the past forty years.

"There is a product commercially known as Sansert. Its generic name is methysergide maleate. It is probably the best preventive medicine you could use in people who have intermittent attacks. It's a derivative of LSD, and sometimes people do have hallucinations with the use of it, but it's rare.

"I have used this drug very effectively without side effects for years. It also is probably the best preventive that you can use for migraine as well. However, if it is used for over six months, steadily, there is a complication that can occur: retroperitoneal fibrosis. In other words, it can stretch the area around the kidney, causing kidney failure, and it can also do that to the lungs, but only with prolonged use. And on rare, very rare occasions, it can cause fibrotic occurrences on the heart valve and lungs.

"When we put a patient on methysergide—we don't use it in migraine; that's number one—we use it in cluster headache, and we never use it for more than three to six months without at least a one- to two-month hiatus in its use. We do six-month and yearly observations of the lungs and chest. We perform tests to make sure we are not getting any side effects. If and when you get any side effects, they are reversible if you stop the drug. The retroperitoneal fibrosis goes away.

"It is probably one of the most valuable drugs we can use for cluster headache. However, a cardiologist wrote an article about one of these rare occurrences in the valves of the heart. And the next thing I knew, there were lawyer ads asking for people taking the drug, or who have ever taken it, obviously looking for business.

"Suddenly, it became unavailable in the U.S. They said they had some manufacturing problems, but it's available from other sources outside the U.S. It's used on such a relatively small number of patients that the market for it is too small to be profitable in the U.S. It was especially worrisome since the lawyers were advertising for them. So they withdrew the product from the U.S. market.

"I used it up until the time I retired, and they still use it in the clinic. We get the drug from Canada.

"I established a rule in the clinic that every prescription was nonrefillable. We practice very careful medicine. It's not done for financial reasons. We're busy enough already. One of the expensive things about doing this is that you have to have a trained person to filter calls for people wanting refills. Usually when the clinic is running, most doctors wouldn't do it, but we had two RNs to listen to patients and cross-reference with their records to assure against any problems with our prescriptions."

Headache care was still very much in the early stages of discovery, and new ideas for treatment were generally well worth a closer look. Among the nonmedicinal treatments Seymour investigated was biofeedback treatment for headaches.

"I'm an avid reader of the *Wall Street Journal,* and they published an article in the early 1970s about the experimental work being done with biofeedback on migraine at the Menninger Clinic in Topeka, Kansas, and on tension headache at the University of Colorado in Boulder. The Menninger Clinic at one time was the largest and best known psychiatric hospital in the United States. The work they were doing—both these institutions—was purely experimental. They were working with patients, but they were feeling their way with it at this time. This was before there was any commercial utilization of instruments to do it. Very grass roots."

Very early work had been done decades ago at the University of Chicago by Dr. Edmund Jacobson, who is recognized as the founder of progressive muscle relaxation and biofeedback. Jacobson, born in 1888, was a doctor of internal medicine and psychiatry and a physiologist as well. He was educated at Northwestern University before going on to Harvard for his M.A. and Ph.D. degrees. He returned to his birthplace, Chicago, where he worked as an assistant in physiology and earned his M.D. degree in 1915. Jacobson had also developed the hardware to read electromyography (EMG) voltages over time, the electrical activity produced by skeletal muscles. He introduced what is now called psychosomatic medicine and was first to accurately measure electrical impulses from muscular contraction, nerves, and mental input at neuromuscular sites in living patients. Now, in Seymour's day, doctors were applying Jacobson's findings to the treatment of headache.

"*The Wall Street Journal* printed a front-page story about people working on a new way to control body functions using Jacobson's autogenic phrases, which are relaxation, self-hypnotic functions. They used medical instruments to illustrate to the patient what happens when they experienced various headache symptoms, and then controlled them by using these autogenic phrases.

"The article discussed the work being done at Menninger Clinic in controlling headaches by Dr. Joseph Sargent, an internist, and two experimental physiologists, Elmer Greene and Dale Walters. It also mentioned the work of Tom Budzinski, Johann Stoyva, and Charles Adler of the University of Colorado in Boulder, in the treatment of biofeedback of headache.

"Because of my specialization and interest in headache, I decided I would be very negligent if I didn't investigate what they were doing. So I called and explained who I was to Dr. Walters at Menninger and arranged a visit to observe their clinical trials and experiments.

"In July of that year, I traveled with two of my nurses, including Mary Franklin, to Topeka, Kansas, and witnessed patients using temperature monitors connected to one of their index fingers while they relaxed. We had the opportunity to speak with a few patients, and I was intrigued. At Menninger, the results in headache were found serendipitously. During experiments with autogenic training, patients were being trained to raise the temperature of their hands. During the process, one of the patients—a migraine sufferer—stopped a headache from continuing.

"Physiology is the study of the workings of the body, and electrophysiologists are concerned with the electrical system of the body. We were very fascinated with their work and their theories on why it worked.

"Then we spent the afternoon with Dr. Joseph Sargent, who was strictly an internist, but presented us about eight to ten of his patients who were successful with the treatments using the instrumentation from Elmer Greene and Dale Walters.

"An interesting aside to this story is that he, like many doctors in that period, lacked the knowledge base for diagnosing headache patients. After he showed us the first two cases and left the room to bring us another case, Mary Franklin said, 'Dr. Diamond, those are cluster headache patients, and they have remissions. Natural remissions.' Even my nurses at that time were more familiar with headache quirks than most doctors. Some of their other cases looked fairly legitimate, even though he was less informed about what or where he was treating. It would never have worked on a cluster headache patient. It's just not the type of disease for that to be responsive.

"In September, we opened our biofeedback department under the supervision of Mary Franklin. We eventually incorporated electro-myographic (EMG) feedback, which had been studied at University of Colorado. It was my opinion that a combination of temperature and EMG biofeedback training would be the best option for our patients. Not every patient was a candidate for biofeedback training, but for those who were open to new techniques, it would be an excellent adjunct to pharmacologic therapy. We also noticed that our youngest patients responded very well to biofeedback training because they enjoyed the machines and did not have prolonged histories of headache which would impact on their responses.

"During the winter of 1974, I presented my first paper on biofeedback and headache at the annual meeting of the Bio-feedback Society of America (now the Association of Applied Psychophysiology and Biofeedback, AAPB), which was held that year in Colorado Springs. In September 1975, I presented further findings at the International College of Psychosomatic Medicine's second symposium of Autogenic Therapy in Rome."

Managed care had denied reimbursement for biofeedback services starting during the early 1980s. Through Seymour's diligence and pressure on the insurance companies, biofeedback training was recognized as an effective therapy. The biofeedback department remained an active area of the clinic as well as the inpatient unit. It is an integral part of the multidisciplinary approach to the hospitalized headache patient. In 2005, Seymour was honored to receive the Presidential Recognition Award of the AAPB, presented by Steve Baskin, Ph.D., who was president of the association at the time.

Acupuncture, an alternative medicine procedure in which needles are inserted and manipulated at certain points on the human body, is claimed by its proponents to relieve pain. It originated in the East, most notably China, where it was first used in conjunction with herbal medicine to treat various illnesses.

As a doctor whose primary purpose was to alleviate headache pain, Seymour had expressed a curiosity in the subject. Then in 1971, *New York Times* journalist James "Scotty" Reston traveled with the media entourage that followed President Richard M. Nixon on his historical trip to China. Reston's story on the resulting experience created a nationwide American interest in the subject.

Reston suffered an appendicitis attack on the trip, and he underwent emergency surgery to remove the appendix at Anti-Imperialist Hospital in Beijing. The operation was conducted successfully using contemporary anesthesia, but it was Reston's postoperative care that captured his—and this country's—imagination. He was treated by Li Chang Yuan using acupuncture, and Reston wrote of his miraculous treatment in a *New York Times* column.

"Suddenly, everybody wanted to know about acupuncture," Seymour recalls. "There was nobody doing acupuncture in the United States. It's prevalent today, but back then, there was no such thing as a registered acupuncturist. I became interested in [its] relationship to headache, whether it would help people or not.

"So I decided I wanted to learn about it. I always had my mind open to it. I didn't want to go to China or anywhere else in the Far East. The only places where they had courses in acupuncture were in France and England.

"During this time, I was asked to give a lecture in La Crosse, Wisconsin, and there I met a neurosurgeon by the name of Norman Shealy. He had just become famous and received a prestigious award from the American Headache Society for some original work about the electrostimulation of the spinal cord to relieve certain painful conditions—not headache—but other painful conditions.

"When I was there I talked to him about acupuncture. He had gone to England about six months prior to see a Dr. Felix Mann, who was probably the guru of teaching acupuncture in the Western World."

Felix Mann, a German-born acupuncturist, devised a system known as Scientific Acupuncture and is the founder and past-president of the Medical Acupuncture Society. He was also the first president of the British Medical Acupuncture Society and the author of the first comprehensive English language acupuncture textbook, *Acupuncture: The Ancient Chinese Art of Healing and How It Works Scientifically.*

"I decided to see what I could learn from Dr. Mann," Seymour says. "He held an intensive two-week course. Elaine and I traveled to London and stayed in a hotel while I studied with Dr. Mann and she explored the city.

"I learned about the points you use for various diseases. I was primarily interested in headache, and he spent almost a day on the treatment of headache with acupuncture. When I came back to Chicago, I did some selective use of it, but it was not consistent with any current medical thinking at that time.

"I was already very much into a different type of medicine with biofeedback, and I didn't want to have too many opinions conflicting with the normal thoughts that were prevalent. And I didn't want to give the impression I was going off the deep end, which could easily be interpreted.

"I used it for about twenty to twenty-five years selectively on certain patients, but the consistency was never great. I really do not believe in it today. I think that a lot of medicine is suggestive."

Like placebos?

"Well, I don't like that word. I prefer 'suggestive.' No matter what therapy you use on certain patients, if they're convinced it's going to work, it's going to help to a certain degree. 'Suggestive' is a good word for it."

Interestingly enough, even Felix Mann no longer supports the practice and has rethought his beliefs in the existence of acupuncture points and meridians. As he states in his book entitled *Reinventing Acupuncture: A New Concept of Ancient Medicine,* "The meridians of acupuncture are no more real than the meridians of geography. If someone were to get a spade and tried to dig up the Greenwich meridian, he might end up in a lunatic asylum. Perhaps the same fate should await those doctors who believe in acupuncture meridians."

In contrast, Dr. Shealy, who retired in 1999, has continued his research into treatments for chronic pain outside of the established medical community. From his website: "[Dr. Shealy] had not been investigating long before he recognized that the majority of long term fixes for chronic pain did not come from the established medical community, but from the 'folk domain.' Shealy began a series of research and experimental processes which included any ideas he could come across that claimed to be able to treat chronic pain in the long term without the use of narcotic medications. Consulting and researching with acupuncturists, mystics, faith healers, color therapists, folk healers, and other non-traditional therapists, and blending this new knowledge with his medical background, Dr. Shealy came to the conclusion that, while none of these methods was *the* cure for chronic pain, almost all of them had developed a documented history of being able to successfully eliminate chronic pain in a good number of their attempts. It is at this juncture that he decided that 'It is the interaction of the four main fields of stress; the chemical, physical, electromagnetic, and emotional; that is the cause of all illness … not some, all.'"

25. Mortality

In Seymour's younger days, he attended an American Medical Association meeting in Atlantic City. He was twenty-seven years old at the time. One of the event's features was the offer of free physical examinations for the attending doctors.

"So I decided to take advantage," Seymour remembers. "They did a cardiogram on me, and it showed that I had a right bundle branch block on the right side of my heart. A thallium stress test, also known as a nuclear stress test, is an imaging method which demonstrates the flow of blood into the heart muscle while you are at rest or during activity (walking on a treadmill). When I underwent this test, it revealed I had decreased circulation to the anterior parts of my heart. Subsequently, angiographs were performed on the coronary arteries (which supply oxygen to the heart). Again, the decreased circulation was evident.

"The heart has its own electrical system, and my later investigations showed that it had no clinical significance in a person my age. I was probably born with it, and it would not affect my lifestyle or longevity."

When Seymour was sixty-four, he experienced four to six episodes of light-headedness. His internist recommended that he undergo a treadmill stress test, and the results were worrisome.

"I reached a heart rate of 129 after one minute," Seymour recalls, "but they had to stop the test because the cardiogram changed. There was a depression in what they call the ST segment, which meant that my coronary arteries were not working right.

"I went to see a cardiologist, Aaron Shafer, who had been doing consults for me at Weiss Hospital. He thought I should have a thallium stress test. That's where they inject a chemical, thallium, into your heart. I took the test, and it showed a lack of circulation to the heart, and the anterior parts of the heart, which was reversible. I then had angiographs done, which showed a questionable constriction of the coronary arteries, the arteries that supply the heart.

"So in consultation with Dr. Shafer, my family, and the people who did the angiograph, I decided that I would have a bypass operation. It's called a CABG, pronounced 'cabbage.'"

The acronym CABG stands for coronary artery bypass graft and is more commonly known as bypass surgery. Arteries from another part of the patient's body are grafted to the coronary arteries, literally bypassing the blocked or narrowed sections, to increase blood flow to the myocardium, or heart muscle.

"There was a choice of various hospitals where I could have the work done. Then, we attended a party with some of our friends, and they introduced me to another friend of theirs who was at the party. (They knew nothing of my condition. I didn't go around advertising it.) We met a charming young woman, probably in her thirties, by the name of Renee Hartz, who happened to sit at the same table. She told me that she was with the cardiac team, a surgeon at Northwestern University.

"Now, doing bypasses is not without risk. In a bypass, they stop the heart, the heart is stopped while they're doing the surgery, and a heart-lung machine (cardiopulmonary bypass pump) takes over until the patient's heart is ready to resume its work. Some people never awaken from it. I knew all the risks, and I felt that it was early in my life, so I decided to undergo the operation. The surgery would be done at Northwestern University Hospital; someone recommended the Cleveland Clinic, but I wanted to do it locally, and now I knew Dr. Hartz, so I saw her and scheduled the surgery.

"I underwent the procedure in December 1989. I've had some heart issues since, but I think it helped me to survive. That's almost twenty-three years. My father had a history of severe angina too.

"I continued seeing Dr. Shafer, who was my cardiologist, until about a year after my surgery when he died. He was about sixty-three at the time, and he died of acute coronary artery disease. Sudden death. We had grown quite close during this time, and they asked me to do the eulogy at his funeral.

"Well, now I had to find another cardiologist. I was on staff at Columbus Hospital at the time, and there I met Nenad Belic, a wonderful cardiologist. He put me on dietary treatment and early medicine to prevent coronary artery disease, much of it before it was recognized by most physicians. He took very good care of me.

"After two or three years, Dr. Belic advised me that he was going to turn me over to one of his colleagues (and he was young, I think he was fifty-six or fifty-seven) because he had a hobby and he wanted to pursue it. And I guess he had all the money in the world. He was married to heiress Ellen Stone, whose family founded J. H. Stones & Sons in 1926. It later became the Stone Container Corporation, a leading manufacturer of paperboard and paper-based packaging.

"He turned me over to my present cardiologist, Perla Benrubi, who has taken care of me wonderfully to this day, even managing my care when I developed a condition requiring a pacemaker.

"On my last visit to Dr. Belic, he said, 'I'm going to row across Lake Michigan. That's my hobby. I like rowing.' And about eight or nine months later, there was a story in the paper about him doing it. He also told me that he was going to contemplate rowing across the Atlantic! And sure enough, he did that, too. Almost."

Chicago Magazine writer Peggy Wolff told of Dr. Belic's fate in an article dated February 25, 2002. The following are excerpts from that story.

Taken by Storm

This is the story of one man's obsession by a dream that probably stretched back to an exotic childhood and drove Nenad Belic to defy the wishes and advice of his family, friends, and colleagues. The quest began on May 11, 2001, from Stage Harbor, in Chatham, Massachusetts, a place they call the "elbow" of Cape Cod. In a twenty-one-foot, custom-designed rowboat with no sail or engine to aid him, Belic began a voyage of 2,580 miles to the Portuguese shore. His goal was to get there before September, when hurricane season hits and the raging storms produce, in the dry terms of naval vocabulary, nonnegotiable waves. At the start, he expected that the crossing would take him one hundred-odd days. It was a journey epic and reckless, admirable, and a bit mad. . . .

For 137 days, Belic had been crossing the sea, facing backwards as he pulled on the oars for up to twelve hours a day, often battling headwinds and facing swells of twenty feet. He had shaved himself bald for the start of his journey, but after four months, his dark, graying hair had grown in. There wasn't an ounce of fat left on his body. . . .

Today, no one knows exactly the ferocity of the weather, but in a six- to eight-hour period of time ... the winds that blew from the North Atlantic towards Ireland on Sunday, September 30th, pushed the waves to rise from around fifteen feet high to around thirty feet. Some observers suspect that a Perfect Storm situation came up, in which two wave jams (waves steep and close together) become bigger and more violent until they meet in a rogue wave: one steep, fifty- or sixty-foot wall of water, avalanching over the boat.

At ten-thirty that night, the Irish Coast Guard and HM Coast Guard Falmouth picked up an EPIRB distress signal from Belic's last position, near 51N 15W, placing him 259 miles west of Bantry Bay, Ireland. The beacon could not have been activated accidentally. Belic would have had to pull the EPIRB off a bracket, flip up a cover switch, reach in, and flip the main switch.

At 11:10 p.m., a Royal Air Force Nimrod aircraft located the beacon's flashing light, then circled the area until an RAF rescue helicopter arrived a few hours later. In darkness, amid gale force winds, the RAF dropped two life rafts. The airmen anticipated finding the boat and the rower, but all they saw was the flashing beacon. There was no sign of a boat or debris.

After 143 days at sea, Lun [his boat] and Belic had vanished.

The EPIRB signal, which was relayed throughout the Coast Guard system, prompted the Great Lakes Coast Guard in Cleveland to call Ellen. It reached her on her cell phone at the Chicago Historical Society, where she was spending that Sunday afternoon. A massive rescue operation had been launched, but if Belic was in the sixty-degree water without a survival suit, he wouldn't survive more than two hours.

Shortly after midnight that night, Ellen felt her body enveloped by a warm, loving presence that held her for a few moments and then was gone. "As if he had come to say goodbye," Ellen says. That same night, their daughter Dara, away at school, had a nightmare that her father had drowned.

Seymour's heart received good care from Dr. Benrubi. He did have a pacemaker installed and is going strong with it today. But there was an even more frightening health issue on his horizon: cancer!

"About nineteen years ago, I was having a burning sensation when urinating. My daughter (Merle, the physician) suggested that I do a PSA."

Here is the National Cancer Institute's explanation of PSA test: Prostate-specific antigen (PSA) is a protein produced by cells of the prostate gland. The PSA test measures the level of PSA in the blood. The doctor takes a blood sample, and the amount of PSA is measured in a laboratory. Because PSA is produced by the body and can be used to detect disease, it is sometimes called a biological marker or a tumor marker.

It is normal for men to have a low level of PSA in their blood; however, prostate cancer or benign (not cancerous) conditions can increase a man's PSA level. As men age, both benign prostate conditions and prostate cancer become more common. The most frequent benign prostate conditions are prostatitis (inflammation of the prostate) and benign prostatic hyperplasia (BPH) (enlargement of the prostate). There is no evidence that prostatitis or BPH causes cancer, but it is possible for a man to have one or both of these conditions and develop prostate cancer as well.

A man's PSA level alone does not give doctors enough information to distinguish between benign prostate conditions and cancer. However, the doctor will take the result of the PSA test into account when deciding whether to check further for signs of prostate cancer.

"So I did the PSA test, and it was slightly elevated. They suggested that I have a digital rectal examination of the prostate. And while doing it, the doctor felt something. He then had a sonogram done on the area and detected that I had multiple cancers of the prostate.

"In consulting, I got several opinions before I decided what to do. Finally I went to a urologist at Northwestern University Hospital. Dr. John Garnett was a man in his thirties, and in all these consultations besides him, they thought I should have a radical prostatectomy. Complete removal of the prostate. I decided to go through the operation.

"There's a test known as the Gleason score. By the severity, the number of lesions, and whether [the cancer] extends into glands or into the capsule, the covering of the prostate, they rate it. And the worst score you can have is a ten.

"Two days after surgery, I was in the hospital, and it was uncomfortable because you're incontinent for a couple days. Basically, surgically, he did a good job because I retained control of my urine, which is one of the side effects, and I still had some sexual potency, which you could lose.

"I knew of all these consequences. About the third day, Elaine and I were sitting in the room. He's coming to make a post-op visit, and he says to me—never on a first-name basis—he says, 'Dr. Diamond, you had a nine on your Gleason score. You'd better get your life in order.' Just like that!

"He walked out of the room, and Elaine and I were just shivering! It's a funny, empty feeling I could never describe. In all the years I was in family practice and even in headache practice, I would never give anybody bad news in that way.

"I want to make a remark that in all the years I've practiced medicine, I've tried to think how the patient will feel from whatever I would say to them. The Hippocratic Oath says you should do no harm. Everyone that graduates from medical school takes that oath, but I don't think it encompasses something else that's very important. I think it should also say, 'Do no harm emotionally,' to the patient. I've told people bad news before, but I've told them in a nicer way, in a way where there was some hope or understanding."

It's chilling news when a physician tells a patient to "get his life in order," but as with every other challenge in his life, Seymour was now ready to contest his death sentence.

"Northwestern is a teaching hospital. They had a residency in urology, and I'm a chatty guy, so I became familiar with one of the residents. They have a big urological service and other urologists besides my surgeon. It's not just one doctor there. They had several groups. I was discussing what I had with this resident, and I asked him, 'Is there anything else I can do?'

"I hadn't had a chance to go and look up alternative therapies. I expected to die in six months or a year as the diagnosis suggested.

"And he said to me, 'You know, there's another group doing a research project on external beam radiation therapy over the area subsequent to surgery.'

"I said to him, 'If it were your father, what would you do?'

"He said, 'Well, they're having some interesting results in very bad cases, but don't say anything. I'm in a residency.' This doctor was in a different group from the one who was caring for me.

"So, I went, not to the group, but to the radiologists who do this special physical measurement—it's like physics, the way they measure and give you the treatments—and after post-op, I took the treatments. It was a series of about fourteen or sixteen [treatments]—very uncomfortable, by the way. You have to drink about a gallon of water before because it protects your other organs while they're doing the radiation. It wasn't a pleasant procedure. Fast, but not pleasant.

"[For] about seven years after my prostatectomy and radiation, I had my PSA measured about every three to four months. Basically the belief is that if the cancer is out of you, you shouldn't have any PSA.

"After about four or five years, my PSA started to rise, very gradually. So, I decided that I should see an oncologist friend, Dr. Gershon Locker, who specializes in prostate disease to get his advice. Dr. Locker took care of me for four or five years before he retired, and then I went to see Dr. Daniel Shevrin, an oncologist at Kellogg Cancer Center in Evanston. They followed my PSA, and what they watch for is, not so much as the rise in it, but the *rate* of rise. If it's 5.2 and next time it's 5.4 and next time it's 5.6, you're not too concerned. But if it's 5.2 and then it becomes 6, and then it becomes 7, that's worrisome.

"My PSA was stable for a while, but it started to rise rapidly, so I undertook some hormone treatment, a drug called Lupron. It's a drug that negates testosterone in your body. I responded to that for a long while, but then I became immune. I've gone through this period in my life where I've been on five different or six different drugs. They control it for a long while, and then we go on to another therapy."

Today, Seymour lives in a somewhat comfortable state of remission. He continues to be tested at regular intervals, carefully monitoring his health as he passes through his mid- to late-eighties.

26. Financial Success

"**M**y proudest achievement in life is the establishment and the pushing forth of the National Headache Foundation into the most important organization for headache sufferers," Seymour says today. "The amount of money the National Headache Foundation donated toward research was about $5–$6 million. For initial grants (we provided the seed money for a lot of people doing headache research), we later received large amounts of money from other sources, so the $5–$6 million generated $50–$60 million over the years.

"My establishment of the Diamond Headache Clinic as a multifaceted, patient-oriented, continuity-type practice was my second greatest achievement along with [a] first acute inpatient hospital unit for headache.

"My original work with histamines, tricyclics, and MAOIs were signature items in my life that because of poor education, overcautiousness, and disbelief aren't integrated into common practice of doctors today."

Seymour Diamond is also an astute businessman. In addition to income received for his medical contributions to the world of headache, he also became a shrewd investor, although, like becoming a doctor, it wasn't anything he'd planned in advance.

"I hadn't considered investing my money. When I first started my practice, I wasn't making any money, so I didn't even think about it. I bought some basic life insurance during those years to protect my family, and that was about it. But after I'd become more successful and the opportunity to put my money to work arose, I decided to give it a try."

Before he'd begun his headache practice, still a family doctor receiving emergency calls from the telephone operators (prior to the establishment of the now familiar 911 service), Seymour accepted a fateful call.

"I took care of a large family. The reason I had them as a family: I was developing my practice in the early years, '51 or '52, and on a Sunday about noon, I received a call from the telephone company. There was a shooting of a child, and the operator gave me the address.

"I sped over there, and there were twin girls. They were about two years old. They were at their grandfather's house, and he kept a gun. A cousin, who was about six to eight years old, found the gun and shot one of the twins in the face. It was an accident; he didn't do it on purpose.

"So, I gathered the child in my arms and carried her to the car with the mother and father and drove them right to the ER at one of my hospitals, where I was on the staff but I didn't really spend a lot of time. Thank God it was in a part of her face that didn't show a lot of scar or anything else. It wasn't a big wound, and it was in one cheek.

"I called a friend of mine, who was one of the great surgeons, Leon Aries, and he came in. We assured the family that everything was going to be all right. We gave the child a tetanus shot, and she went home. These people were very gracious, and I started to take care of the whole family. They were nice people, they had a lot of friends, and it really stirred my practice. I hadn't done a lot. I was just there and helped them get some help. I was no hero, maybe a hero to them, but not to anybody else.

"Anyway, one of the relatives of this family came to me as a patient. And he sees a young doctor and he tells me 'I've got a wonderful investment for you.' He tells me he's opening a large car wash, which there weren't many [of] during those days. I'm talking about a really large one. He said he's got eighteen or twenty investors, and he asked if I'd like to become a member. He appeared as though he was being gracious, so I said, 'Fine.' And by the way, I never made an investment after that where I didn't have my own control, all right? And it might be good philosophy for anyone.

"To me, it was a lot of money. I think about $10,000, but that was a lot of money back then. So, the car wash gets built, and I think to myself, 'Well, I'm going to take my car in and get it washed.'

"He was there, and I told him I'd like to have them wash my car, but they wanted to charge me for it!" Seymour laughs. "I was offended, but I paid. He said, 'The policy is we don't give any courtesy washes to anybody.'

"So, time passes, and I talked to him several times about returns on my investment, but he would say, 'It's growing, but we've got a big investment, and we can't take anything out yet.'

"Then, on a July afternoon, I went out to play golf with some friends. We got to the ninth hole, when somebody told me Elaine had called for me. I called her back, and she told me that the car wash owner had called, and he said it was urgent for me to call him.

"I called him, and he said to me, 'You know, Seymour, you're a partner in this, and I want to do something for you. I want to simonize and detail your car for you, as a courtesy.' I left the golf course, and it really bothered me. Why would this guy, all of a sudden, offer me what he'd denied me before?

"I called him the next day, and in the contract I signed, it said that I could withdraw within a certain number of months if I wanted to. And I said to him, 'You know, I'd like my money back.'

"He said to me, 'Well, we can't do that.'

So, I said, 'Maybe we should have a meeting with the other investors to see how they feel about letting me out, giving me my money.' I had a list of everybody that was involved.

But he said, 'Oh no, don't do that. I'll send you a check.'

"He sent me a check. It bounced three times, and then finally on the fourth attempt, it was good. And I was out. And about three months later, the car wash went bankrupt. It was a valuable lesson for a new investor."

Seymour's next investment would be his partnership with Leroy Jorgensen, the electrical supply store owner, and David Sachs, a lighting fixture manufacturer, when they worked with Verne Oscarson to build three medical structures. One of them housed the Diamond Headache Clinic. The others are the properties Seymour owned and leased to other doctors, earning a satisfying return on his investment, until he realized that being a landlord wasn't for him.

While constructing the buildings, one of the subcontractors, a plasterer named Steve Mestan, let it be known that he owned an oil well in Iowa, and he asked if Seymour was interested in becoming an investor.

"It was pumping oil," Seymour relates. "It did bring me dividends. I didn't have control over it, but there were enough people I knew who were partners in this venture, and I got more than my investment out of it.

"I flew out one time with Steve, and he was a bit of a playboy, although I didn't realize it at the time. We went to the airport, and he says, 'I've gotta buy some insurance.'

"I said, 'OK, maybe I should buy some, too.' That was the time everybody was afraid of flying, and they bought airline life insurance from booths that were found in every airport. It's not like that anymore, of course.

"So I took out a policy for Elaine. I saw him in there, and he was doing about ten different policies. So in the plane I said, 'Steve, why do you do all those policies?'

"And he replied, 'Well, you know, I'm not married, and I've got a lot of girlfriends. I buy a policy for each of them, and when they ask me why, I tell them if anything happened to me, I'd want to know that they were taken care of.'"

Not all of Seymour's investments provided a good return, and here Seymour tells us about one of the odder ones.

"Marv Cohn [Seymour's lawyer friend] and I went into a very interesting one. I brought him into it, I'm ashamed to say. I had a patient who was a full professor at one of the universities in biology and aquatic sciences.

"That professor had the idea—and this is before anyone else was doing this—of how to raise shrimp on a farm. He proposed going to Thailand, where you could get these made cheaply, like little lakes or pools to raise shrimp. Marv and I were interested. We pooled our money and financed it, which was a big mistake.

"It was about 1978 and Klausmeyer was intrigued about doing it. Looking at it in retrospect, he wasn't a good enough businessman to do something like that. It seemed like a good idea because that was before people were doing it. We'd be the first.

"Klausmeyer set it up, but it never made any money. He had trouble doing marketing. He called me years later and said, 'I'm going to pay you back for helping me.' I had some stock issues he made. But I still have the stock issues and no return on my investment. Finally, I stopped hearing from him."

It wasn't until the early 1980s that Seymour began investing in the stock market, and as with almost everything else in his life, that opportunity arose through the dealings of a grateful patient.

"In 1982, I saw a man named Walter Wilson from the Baltimore area. He had cluster headaches, and I was able to help him. On one of his visits—he flew in about three times a year to see me—he said to me, 'Seymour, what are you doing about investing?'

"I had no concept of stock or anything else at that point.

"He said, 'You know, I'm the head of this stock company in this office, W. H. Newbolds, and I'd like to help you in your investments. I give you my word that if you take any losses, I will repay you personally.'

"That was my first association with the stock market. And he did very well. I mean, I wasn't a big investor, but he took care that I made good money on my investments and they were safe.

"In 1990, they were sold, and Walter had retired in about 1988. He gave me over to a young stockbroker named Chuck McKain, and Chuck moved over to Legg Mason with the sale, and I went with him. Legg Mason later became Smith Barney and then Morgan Stanley. Chuck and his partner David Metz still manage my portfolio today.

"And they have been wonderful in helping me with both my retirement and other investments through the years."

Seymour's other investments have been in the form of housing for Elaine and himself. In addition to their Chicago apartment, they also own a condominium in Palm Springs, California.

First came the Palm Springs condominium. Seymour was lecturing at the Universal City Hilton in Los Angeles, Elaine was with him, and they decided to add a couple of vacation days to their stay. Seymour's stepbrother Al, who was also a doctor and lived in Los Angeles, made them an offer.

"We were in Los Angeles for a meeting," Elaine recalls, "and his brother called. He said, 'I have a place in Palm Springs that we bought as an investment.' Somebody had opened a whole area of new condos called Andreas Hills, and one of his friends had bought one. He and his wife bought one, too. Supposedly, they would use it to come down for a weekend, rarely, but more as an investment. So he called Seymour and said, 'We're not using it, so why don't you go stay at it for the weekend instead of staying at a hotel?'

"We agreed to try it. But the day before we were supposed to go—this was at the beginning of the weekend—he called, very excited because he had a chance to rent it for four months. That was part of the idea on this investment, to rent it out. So, Seymour said, 'Not a problem, we'll stay at a hotel down there, and it'll be fine.'

"So we rented a car and started driving down Interstate 10 toward Palm Springs. It was not a nice day; it was misty and gray with a light rain, and we said, 'Oh, this could be nothing, but we'll try it.'

"And as we got closer to Palm Springs—you know … those drawings the kids make where there's a yellow circle with the little beams coming out of it, like the sun? That's what I saw. And I said, 'Seymour, that has to be Palm Springs!' In the midst of all this gray, misty rain, there was this yellow circle of the sun shining down, and it turned out to be a gorgeous weekend!

"We stayed at the old Canyon Hotel, which was a favorite among movie stars. It's no longer there. Long gone. But it was [a] small hotel, very Hollywood, it had a winding stairway, and a wonderful singer in the bar, and we had a great weekend! We enjoyed it, and that was our first trip to Palm Springs.

"The following year," Elaine continues, "Seymour asked his brother if there was anyone who could rent us a house. His brother talked to a real estate lady who lived in the area, and she found somebody who would rent us a place for a month. It was a two-story and very nice. We did that for one month, and the following year we did it again, and by the third year, we rented for two months and started looking for a place. Nobody believed Seymour would do it, but there was FedEx and there was fax to keep him in touch with Chicago. It didn't have all the conveniences, but there was FedEx and fax, so we did it."

Seymour's brother's house was in Andreas Hills, a nice section with a sign that proclaimed it to be "the Bel Air of Palm Springs." It was quiet, secluded, away from the bustle of the city's main thoroughfare, Highway 111, up against the hills.

"The area's kind of funny," Seymour picks up the story. "There are five groups of condos in the areas, and they're surrounded by $1 million to $5 million homes. It was up in the hills, which is beautiful.

"We met this real estate woman who was very aggressive, Zelda Segal," he continues. "She showed us this house. It was owned by a decorator. When it was built, she put in lots of upgrades. We made an offer. She counteroffered, and we bought the place. Very happily, we bought the place. We bought some of her furniture, too.

"Zelda and her husband Manny befriended us. They lived in a gigantic mansion with an Olympic-sized swimming pool and their own tennis court. At the time, she was known as the one who'd sold the biggest property in Palm Springs, and she was interviewed by *60 Minutes* for that one. And that's how we wound up buying a home in Palm Springs."

As the children grew and left home, Seymour and Elaine's Springfield Avenue home back in Evanston seemed to get bigger and bigger. Eventually, they decided to move again, this time to a condominium in downtown Chicago.

"We lived in the Skokie-Evanston area, the children had left already, and it was a big house. Some of our friends moved downtown, but I wasn't ready yet. Then, one day I said to Elaine, 'Let's look around.' And we started to look at different condominiums.

"A lot of them were really overpriced in comparison to the house we lived in. These people wanted a lot for the same space. But, finally, a very nice real estate agent took us into the Carlisle here, where we live today.

"We saw an apartment we liked, and they were asking close to a million dollars for it! There were a lot nicer ones and lot of worse ones, but this was the one we really liked.

"I said, 'Boy, I wish we could buy it!'

"Elaine said, 'Well, I don't like the chandelier in front of the building anyway.' (They have a big, old-fashioned chandelier. It sort of sets it off. I like it!)

"Then the real estate woman called me back and she said, 'Dr. Diamond, do you want to make an offer on it?'

"I said, 'There's a big difference between what I can offer and what they're asking. Wouldn't it be a foolish effort?'

"And she said to me, 'Well, it never hurts to make an offer.'

"So, I made an offer for less than half of what they were asking. And next thing I know, they counteroffered about $300,000 lower than their original asking price. They wanted to get out, they had some problems, or they wouldn't have come down like that.

"I stood pretty firm because I didn't want to pay more than $450,000 for it. That's what I could afford.

"But we finally settled at $506,000, and that's how we bought the apartment. We've been here ever since! We couldn't have had anything better than what we have here. Nice neighbors, all the services we ever wanted. It's just great. It was a great move."

In wrapping up the chapter on his financial prowess, Seymour adds, "I believe my early experience in managing my investments served me well later on when I became responsible for managing the Diamond Headache Clinic and the National Headache Foundation."

27. Retirement

"In 2007, I was eighty-two years old. Elaine and I talked it over, and we decided that we would like to step out—I would like to step out of the practice. Retire.

"I had tried many times during the previous years to use outside management people, and what I mean by 'outside' is hiring a manager for the practice. But really it never worked out. Between Mary Franklin and me, with her help, we had taken care of management very adequately, even through the rougher years when I started the headache practice, and worked through it.

"But times had changed. I had four partners and over fifty employees. I was the majority partner. I thought it would be very easy for me to just step out without them paying me vast sums even though the practice itself is valuable and the name has tremendous worth. It was the first private headache clinic in the country, and to this day, we still get referrals from all over the world.

"I had Jim Staulcup, my personal lawyer, start negotiating. They had a lawyer also, and it happened to be Merle's lawyer, a friend of hers.

"There was tremendous discussion going on between Jim and the other lawyer. He would come up with one idea, but then her lawyer would come up with another. It was a difficult negotiation, and it lasted two years! I lost two years of my life that I wanted to spend in other ways.

"At the end, when it all got finalized, I practically wanted to give it away by that time, but I came out much better than I thought I would. Not a lot of money, but better than I'd anticipated. There were four lawyers involved, one for each partner."

Jim Staulcup, longtime friend, patient, and counsel to Seymour offers his own perspective on the negotiations: "Since Seymour has told me to talk about it, I can do that. We would be at the point where we thought we had a resolution, and Seymour would change his mind. So there was some of that. It was a difficult negotiation because on the one hand, I'm the attorney for the clinic, which is a corporate entity, and on the other, I'm the attorney for the major shareholder, Seymour. The first thing we told him is that, although Merle had her own attorney, the two other shareholders should have their own attorneys in the negotiations. I couldn't represent the major shareholder and the corporate entity, and that was fine. But that also tossed four attorneys into the pot.

"They did retain their own attorneys, and I brought in another attorney, Coco Soodek. Caroline's her first name, but everyone calls her Coco. I told her I've been working primarily in labor and employment, and I can negotiate. I'm used to negotiating. But there are a lot of tricky things here in terms of corporate issues and setting forth so that there is no appearance that there's pressure involved here. I told Seymour I was going to stand on the side. I would overview everything, and Coco would do the rest of the negotiations.

"And so, for the last year of the negotiation, I kind of was on the sidelines, overseeing it. There were things that would come in that Coco wouldn't understand, and I'd help then.

"The others had attorneys, and they had questions, and when you're dealing with three other parties, it just adds another element—explanation—because one of the parties understands how things are done, but another doesn't, and so you have to go through all of that. But it was worked out to Seymour's satisfaction. I think it was June 27, 2007 (I don't know why the date sticks in my mind), that all the documents were signed and executed. And then Seymour retired in 2008.

"And, again, they agreed to some things that he wanted, such as the valuation of his interest and the like. They took it to their attorneys, and they all agreed. I would have had a new appraisal done of the value of the shares of stock because I think it would have been lower than what he ended up with. It was just a very tedious process.

"The last year, it was mostly Coco's doing and not mine. I just would prompt her with certain things, give her some background, but let her deal with the other attorneys. She did a good job."

Seymour continues, "I guess the attitudes of younger physicians are different today. I know what I went through when I built a practice, how hard it was for me. Now, these kids get out of school; they get a job; they don't have to establish anything. It was a different world back then, and I really want to make a distinction in the book about it.

"I always had a policy in the office that it was kept open on Saturdays. We alternated, but everybody took a turn working on Saturdays. First of all, it was a source of increased revenue for the practice. Second, it was a convenience, especially to the numerous out-of-town patients and working people who couldn't come in during the week. They could come to see us without leaving their employment. It was a wonderful thing to do for people!

"But with lobbying and threats, I was forced to give up the Saturday thing a couple years before my retirement negotiation. We ran a very high overhead; we had over fifty employees, which affected the overall finances of the practice.

"Back then, we started with four weeks' vacation, but they wanted six weeks. Under pressure, I gave them that. Sick days became more frequent, too.

"Another occurrence happened in 1999 or 2000. I had always, in all my speeches, in all my talking—when I started the practice I used to do as many as one hundred talks a year—but I never neglected the practice because of it. Never. I always tried to arrange my date ... on a weekend or a date when I wouldn't be in the office anyway. I had a policy of expecting minor gifts or small amounts of money as an honorarium for my talks.

"The same sort of thing occurred with this; the partners wanted to give talks. We counted the days off as establishing the credence of the practice. I thought it was important for us to get out, for people to know us, especially doctors. I'm talking about lecturing to other doctors. I never lectured in a restaurant or other places; I always lectured within a hospital or academic institution in all those years.

"However, in the late 1990s through today, the industry became interested in having sponsoring speakers. The speakers wouldn't specifically mention their product, but then there would be a luncheon or dinner sponsored by the pharmaceutical company to promote their products.

"One of the partners began to take excessive amounts of days off for speaking out of the office and not making them up. And of course, the policy was that they could keep the money and they could have time off. But one partner abused it and another partner felt, 'If this partner can do it, then I can do it,' and it became a magnified abuse.

"It actually became a situation where they were working for the pharmaceutical industry more than they were working for us while they were drawing their salaries! Then they started to compete, to determine which partner could do the most pharmaceutical talks.

"This and the other things were some of my reasons for wanting to leave. It wasn't any fun anymore. We had some difficult management issues that weren't about medicine. It was just ugly.

"I tried to talk to them about the reality of what they were doing, but the only thing I received back was threats. If I had been twenty years younger, I wouldn't have had any qualms of getting rid of at least two of the ones who were abusing it.

"During this period, I kept up my participation in the practice. I wasn't taking days off. I did what I could. But finally, I decided, after we got that contract done, I would phase out my practice.

"Over a two-year period, I referred my patients to other physicians in the practice. I had a fairly close relationship with the majority of my patients, and I tried to very carefully give them out to doctors who I thought would conscientiously take care of them.

"There were four partners at that time, besides myself. I held a majority stake in the practice; I had 51 percent. My lawyers, thank God, wouldn't let me give away any more. And I had given them their partnerships without charging any of them. When they became partners, they didn't have to buy their share of the practice; I gave it to them. And at that time, we had tremendous receivables.

"In the meanwhile, I was still seeing patients and phasing out the practice. I thought I would do it for another year. I was disassociated as far as running the clinic. I'm telling you about the 'hurts' in life.

"And while I was in California during the winter—the four months I take off at that time—they moved the office! No, don't laugh! I mean, they were entitled to. This was after the contract, and they could do what they wanted. They moved it to a nice location.

"I came back in May to start seeing patients again, and I went to the new location, but there was no office for me! I've always believed that every doctor should have a private office besides the area where he's seeing patients. I established that policy when I started the practice.

"One of the partners said, 'We want to share an office with you.' So, I decided that maybe we'll finish up this October. I'm through.

"All this time, I was seeing patients, by the way, and I did not collect a salary. I let all the money go into the practice. It wasn't in the contract, and I was phasing out patients, but they were making a lot of money from me seeing these people. I just was trying to phase this out as nice as I could.

"One of the things that really irritated me is that nobody even took me out to lunch. No retirement celebration of any type. Nothing.

"Dr. Freitag called me two days after I left and said he would like to have a gathering at his house. He told me that nothing was formally done at the office because of the opposition of one of the partners. And then, about a year later, Dr. Urban asked to do it. I guess he had talked it over with the other partners, and this time, they all agreed to do it. But I said, 'No, thank you.'

"After I left the practice, I decided I would spend my time helping the National Headache Foundation. I moved over there and was able to get millions of dollars of grants for them. I have a nice office over there. It's gratifying that I was able to work for an organization that was doing so much good for headache people.

"The last part of this whole thing is that when I quit, I still had a separate foundation, the Diamond Research & Educational Foundation that I established and had funded all these years. I did educational meetings, and I drew a small salary. It belonged to me, and I had complete control. I didn't leave it with them. It was a lot of work, and I ran a big meeting in Palm Springs, another one in Disney World down in Florida, and one in Chicago.

"It was something that took some of my time, but I ran it very well, Mary Franklin and myself. Then, all of a sudden, I get a lawyer who was hired by an individual trying to take my foundation back for the practice. They were accusing me of all types of machinations, actually short of calling me a crook. So I decided to divorce myself from the whole thing."

Finally officially retired, Seymour expresses his appreciation for one of his most meaningful acknowledgements.

"There had been many discussions about how to honor my legacy in headache medicine. One suggestion was the establishment of a chair in headache at one of the medical schools, but I especially liked the idea of a fellowship in my name, in which a physician from any discipline would be able to study at a headache center for one year and learn the various aspects of headache under the tutelage of a headache specialist.

"In October 1993, the National Headache Foundation honored me with a tribute. The proceeds would be the seed money for the Seymour Diamond, M.D. Fellowship in Headache Medicine. There were close to three hundred guests, and it felt like my adult 'bar mitzvah.' The important result was that we could initiate the fellowship program.

"The first Seymour Diamond, M.D. Headache Fellow was Lisa Mannix, M.D. Lisa completed her fellowship at the Cleveland Clinic under the watchful eyes of my friends and colleagues, Robert Kunkel and Glen Solomon. As would be required by all of the fellows, Lisa presented a lectureship at one of the postgraduate courses that we sponsored. She later started her own headache clinic, outside of Cincinnati, and became a member of the board of the NHF.

"For the next few years, the applications were limited, and we saw the need for the fellowship to be certified by one of the specialty boards. I also wanted the Diamond Headache Clinic methods imparted to these fellows, providing them with clinical experience at the outpatient center, as well as the Diamond Inpatient Headache Unit at Saint Joseph Hospital in Chicago. This unit is the largest private inpatient unit in the U.S., with thirty-six inpatient beds and a multidisciplinary staff.

"With the help of Doctors José Biller and Rima Dafer of the Department of Neurology at Loyola University Chicago Stritch School of Medicine, a one-year fellowship program was approved by the United College of Neurologic Specialties. The fellow would complete the program at Loyola and the Diamond Headache Clinic.

"We received many applications from physicians who had completed approved residences in neurology, internal medicine, and family medicine. In July 2010, the first fellow in the approved program, Sandra Pinilla, M.D., began her work at the clinic and at Loyola. I was especially delighted because Sandra had just completed her residency in family practice. She presented her lecture at our Palm Springs course in February 2011 and is now on the staff of the Diamond Headache Clinic. For the years 2012 through 2013, there will be two fellows completing the program at the Clinic and at Loyola.

"The importance of this fellowship is to train physicians in the nuances of headache management. It also serves to broadcast the importance of training in headache medicine and that it involves many disciplines. I am very honored to have this fellowship named for me, and I could not find a better mentor for these fellows than my good friend, José Biller, who is head of Loyola's Department of Neurology.

"Because of the Diamond Headache Clinic Research & Educational Foundation, which supports the program, we have also provided travel grants to residents and newly practicing physicians to attend the postgraduate courses in Palm Springs and Orlando. These physicians are exposed to the various headache issues and the management complexities of headache disorders."

In October 2011, Elaine was involved in a horrific accident when her car collided with a truck on the streets of Chicago. Emergency help responded, and she was hospitalized in the intensive care unit at Illinois Masonic Hospital.

"I didn't know how much Elaine meant to me until she had the accident," Seymour tells us today. "You know, you never really realize it. It's often said that once a wife goes, a husband goes soon after. I was a total loss mentally and physically during that period. I thought the whole world had disintegrated."

The incident was also tinged with a sense of déjà vu. Seymour's father, Nathan Diamond, had endured a similar experience.

"Two years before his death, he had an automobile accident; actually, he hit a parked car. Déjà vu! He came to me and told me about it, so I left my patients and went over. I found out whose car it was and told them I would take care of everything and please don't worry about it."

Nathan, fortunately, wasn't badly hurt in the incident. Elaine, however, was another case entirely.

"She had a subdural brain hemorrhage, which thankfully receded by itself. She would have needed brain surgery, but it started to recede. We watched it. The hospital neurosurgeons saw it first on the CAT scan, and they followed it. When it didn't expand or spread, we knew it was going away. But it was touch-and-go. She also fractured her orbit, multiple ribs, her femur, and her patella. She had bad injuries, and it was touch-and-go for the first three days. I slept there every night. I wanted to be near her.

"She previously had hip replacements—the last one was about four or five years ago. With the femur fracture, normally they put a shaft in to stabilize it, and the patient can start mobility right away. But having the hip operation destroyed that option. They had to fasten the broken bone externally. Not outside of the skin, but to operate and fasten it together with screws and wires rather than having just a steel rod inserted.

"One interesting thing: To make the bone grow faster and to stabilize it, they put in a cadaver's fibula, a bone transplant. The fibula is the small bone that stabilizes the knee and the ankle. I never heard of them doing that in repairing a fracture, so I was a little shocked to hear they attached a fibula on the side of her femur to encourage the healing.

"The accident happened October 14, and her surgery was on October 17. The delay was caused by the fact that she was on blood thinners. She had suffered a small stroke about ten years ago, so she was on blood thinners for that, and they couldn't take a chance on doing the surgery at that time.

"As far as the cause of the accident is concerned, I didn't ask her about it for two months. And she didn't say anything to me. They issued her a ticket, but it was dismissed in court. She didn't appear, but Nate [son-in-law Nathan Diamond-Falk] had somebody appear for her.

"Anyway, she's got a wonderful attitude. You know, she's going to be eighty-five a week after I'm eighty-seven in 2012, and a lot of people would have given up. But she's doing intensive physical therapy. He comes in three times a week, and she does her exercises. And they're painful, too!"

Elaine's accident frightened us all. She's recovering steadily, taking her time to do everything her doctor advises, exactly as prescribed. But it's apparent that the incident was a real eye-opener for them. It was a close call. Any slight variation in the crash could have made matters much worse. We were scared. We came close to losing her, and that sobering fact makes us appreciate her determined fight to recover all the more.

In this sixth week of 2012, almost four months since the accident, Elaine has recovered to the point where she's mobile again. She uses a cane for security, but now she can return to normal life with its restaurant dinners, bridge tournaments, and family affairs.

"My and Elaine's personal relationship with our daughters—Judi Diamond-Falk and her husband Nathan, Merle who is now in charge of the clinic, and Amy with her husband Charlie—is attentive and exemplary. Elaine and I are the proud grandparents of six wonderful young adults. Judi and Nathan's son Brian Diamond-Falk works in the culinary field and lives in Maine with his wife Katie, who is an internal medicine and pediatric specialist. Brian's sister Emily is in Washington, D.C. where she and her husband Alex work at the Pew Institute. Merle's oldest son Max, a recent law school graduate, is in practice in Chicago doing civil rights law. Michael, an investment banker and financial analyst, is working in Dallas, Texas. Her son Jacob recently graduated from Wesleyan University in hopes of pursuing a career in psychology. And daughter Katelynn is finishing high school in Virginia. We are also proud and fortunate to have two great-grandchildren from Brian and Katie's marriage. Zevon, a darling five-year-old girl named after musician Warren Zevon, and Oliver, an overactive treasure. We communicate weekly by Skype."

For Seymour, retirement with his now-healthy life partner is finally going well again.

"I enjoy every day. Part of the secret is that I have a good marriage. We are basically similar and share the same basic values and goals. And I'd say that we have an abiding friendship at this point, an example being that we enjoy mysteries on television. We only enjoy playing bridge as partners—it's very rare that people play strictly as a partner or husband and wife. We do have arguments at the table or immediately after we finish playing, but it's all forgotten once we get home.

"I think it's important that I selected a career that gives me some prestige, and I enjoyed what I was doing all through my years with the Diamond Headache Clinic. Now, I'm enjoying going into work at the National Headache Foundation, not on a daily basis, but more as an advisor, and I'm able to do a service there.

"I think it's terrible that people do things that they're unhappy with. You can't deny your true passions, and you should pursue the career you want. Life is too short not to. I've been involved in something that I absolutely love. I've been fortunate that, although it was not my main objective, by pure chance I got into the headache world. And it's been a tremendous experience for me.

"I took advantage of all the opportunities I had and the challenges, and I think that's important. I've adopted a policy of being happy. Every day is a good day for me, and I look forward to it!"

As he has done in each of his thousands of lectures, Seymour ends his book with a quotation by the Chicago journalist Sydney J. Harris:

A bad doctor treats symptoms.
A good doctor treats ailments.
A rare doctor treats patients.